ABC of
COPD

Second Edition

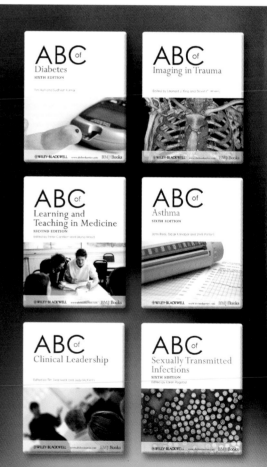

ABC of

COPD

Second Edition

EDITED BY

Graeme P. Currie

Consultant in Respiratory and General Medicine
Aberdeen Royal Infirmary
Aberdeen, UK

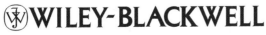

WILEY-BLACKWELL

A John Wiley & Sons, Ltd., Publication

BMJ|Books

Library of Congress Cataloging-in-Publication Data

ABC of COPD / edited by Graeme P. Currie. – 2nd ed.
     p. ; cm. – (ABC series)
  Includes bibliographical references and index.
  ISBN 978-1-4443-3388-6
  1. Lungs – Diseases, Obstructive. I. Currie, Graeme P. II. Series: ABC series (Malden, Mass.)
  [DNLM: 1. Pulmonary Disease, Chronic Obstructive. WF 600]
  RC776.O3A23 2011
  616.2′4 – dc22

                                                    2010029198

A catalogue record for this book is available from the British Library.

This book is published in the following electronic formats: ePDF 9781444329476; ePub 9781444329483

Set in 9.25/12 Minion by Laserwords Private Limited, Chennai, India
Printed in Singapore by Ho Printing Singapore Pte Ltd

1   2011

Contents

Contributors

Peter J. Barnes

Professor of Respiratory Medicine
Airway Disease Section
National Heart and Lung Institute
Imperial College London
London, UK

David Bellamy

Bournemouth General Practitioner (retired)
Bournemouth, UK

John Britton

Professor of Epidemiology
UK Centre for Tobacco Control Studies
University of Nottingham;
Consultant in Respiratory Medicine
City Hospital
Nottingham, UK

Mahendran Chetty

Consultant in Respiratory Medicine
Aberdeen Royal Infirmary
Aberdeen, UK

Graeme P. Currie

Consultant in Respiratory and General Medicine
Aberdeen Royal Infirmary
Aberdeen, UK

Graham S. Devereux

Professor of Respiratory Medicine
Division of Applied Health Sciences
University of Aberdeen;
Consultant in Respiratory Medicine
Aberdeen Royal Infirmary
Aberdeen, UK

Graham Douglas

Consultant in Respiratory Medicine
Aberdeen Royal Infirmary
Aberdeen, UK

Cathy Jackson

Professor of Primary Care Medicine;
Director of Clinical Studies
Bute Medical School
University of St Andrews
St Andrews, UK

Gordon Linklater

Consultant in Palliative Care Medicine
Roxburghe House
Aberdeen, UK

Brian J. Lipworth

Professor of Allergy and Respiratory Medicine
Asthma and Allergy Research Group
Ninewells Hospital and Medical School
Dundee, UK

William MacNee

Professor of Respiratory and Environmental Medicine
MRC Centre for Inflammation Research
Queen's Medical Research Institute
University of Edinburgh
Edinburgh, UK

Paul K. Plant

Consultant in Respiratory Medicine
St James's University Hospital
Leeds, UK

Jadwiga A. Wedzicha

Professor of Respiratory Medicine
Royal Free and University College Medical
School
University College
London, UK

Foreword

Chronic obstructive pulmonary disease (COPD) is a major global epidemic. It already is the fourth commonest cause of death in high income countries and is predicted to soon become the third commonest cause of death worldwide. In the United Kingdom, the mortality from COPD in women now exceeds that from breast cancer. COPD is also predicted to become the fifth commonest cause of chronic disability, largely because of the increasing levels of cigarette smoking in developing countries in conjunction with an ageing population. It now affects approximately 10% of men and women over 40 years in the United Kingdom and is one of the commonest causes of hospital admission. Because of this, COPD has an increasing economic impact, and direct healthcare costs now exceed those of asthma by more than threefold. Despite these startling statistics, COPD has been relatively neglected and is still underdiagnosed in primary care settings. This is in marked contrast to asthma, which is now recognised and well managed in the community. The new NHS National Strategy seeks to improve diagnosis and management of COPD in the community and reduce hospital admissions.

Highly effective treatment is now available for asthma, which has in turn transformed patients' lives. Sadly, this is not the case with COPD, where management is less effective and no drug has so far been shown to convincingly slow progression of the disease. However, we do now have effective bronchodilators and non-pharmacological treatments, which can improve the quality of life of patients. Many patients, however, are not diagnosed or undertreated, so increased awareness of COPD is needed. There are advances in understanding the underlying inflammatory disease, so this may lead to more effective use of existing treatment and the development of new drugs in the future. In this second edition of the *ABC COPD* monograph, Graeme Currie and colleagues provide a timely update on the pathophysiology, diagnosis, and modern management of COPD. It is vital that COPD is recognised and treated appropriately in general practice where the majority of patients are managed, and this book provides a straightforward overview of the key issues relating to this important condition.

Peter J. Barnes FRS, FMedSci
Head of Respiratory Medicine
National Heart & Lung Institute
Imperial College London
London, UK

CHAPTER 1

Definition, Epidemiology and Risk Factors

Graham S. Devereux

Division of Applied Health Sciences, University of Aberdeen, Aberdeen, UK *and*
Aberdeen Royal Infirmary, Aberdeen, UK

OVERVIEW

- Chronic obstructive pulmonary disease (COPD) is characterised by largely irreversible airflow obstruction and an abnormal inflammatory response within the lungs

- It is the fourth leading cause of death in the United States and Europe

- Cases of known COPD are likely to only represent the 'tip of the iceberg' with as many individuals undiagnosed

- Other conditions also cause progressive airflow obstruction and these need to be differentiated from COPD

- COPD is usually caused by cigarette smoking, but pipe, cigar and passive smoking, indoor and outdoor air pollution, occupational exposures, previous tuberculosis and repeated early life respiratory tract infections have all been implicated in its development

- The prevalence of COPD in never smokers (estimated to be between 25 and 45% worldwide) is higher than previously thought; the use of biomass fuel (mainly in developing countries) is one of the main risk factors

Definition

Chronic obstructive pulmonary disease (COPD) is a progressive disease characterised by airflow obstruction and destruction of lung parenchyma. The current definition as suggested by the American Thoracic and European Respiratory Societies is as follows:

COPD is a preventable and treatable disease state characterised by airflow limitation that is not fully reversible. The airflow limitation is usually progressive and associated with an abnormal inflammatory response of the lungs to noxious particles or gases, primarily caused by cigarette smoking. Although COPD affects the lungs, it also produces significant systemic consequences.

COPD is the preferred term for the airflow obstruction associated with the diseases of chronic bronchitis and emphysema (Box 1.1). A number of other conditions are associated with poorly reversible airflow obstruction – for example, cystic fibrosis, bronchiectasis

and obliterative bronchiolitis. These conditions need to be considered in the differential diagnosis of obstructive airway disease, but are not conventionally covered by the definition of COPD. Although asthma is defined by variable airflow obstruction, there is evidence that the airway remodelling processes associated with asthma can result in irreversible progressive airflow obstruction that fulfils the definition for COPD. Because of the high prevalence of asthma and COPD, these conditions co-exist in a sizeable proportion of individuals resulting in diagnostic uncertainty.

Box 1.1 **Definitions of conditions associated with airflow obstruction**

- COPD is characterised by airflow obstruction. The airflow obstruction is usually progressive, not reversible and does not change markedly over several months. The disease is predominantly caused by smoking.
- Chronic bronchitis is defined as the presence of chronic productive cough on most days for 3 months, in each of 2 consecutive years, in a patient in whom other causes of productive cough have been excluded.
- Emphysema is defined as abnormal, permanent enlargement of the distal airspaces, distal to the terminal bronchioles, accompanied by destruction of their walls and without obvious fibrosis.
- Asthma is characterised by reversible, widespread and intermittent narrowing of the airways.

Epidemiology

Prevalence

The prevalence of COPD varies considerably between epidemiological surveys. While this reflects the variation in the prevalence of COPD between and within different countries, differences in methodology, diagnostic criteria and analytical techniques undoubtedly contribute to disparities between studies.

The lowest estimates of prevalence are usually based on self-reported or doctor-confirmed COPD. These estimates are usually 40–50% of the prevalence rates derived from spirometric

ABC of COPD, 2nd edition.
Edited by Graeme P. Currie. © 2011 Blackwell Publishing Ltd.

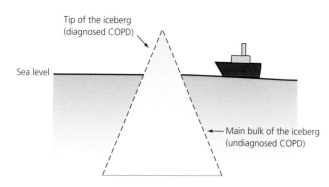

Figure 1.1 Known cases of COPD may represent only the 'tip of the iceberg' with many cases currently undiagnosed.

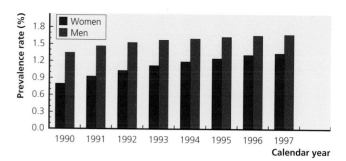

Figure 1.3 Prevalence of diagnosed COPD in UK men and women (per 1000) between 1990 and 1997. Reproduced with permission from Soriano JB, Maier WC, Egger P, *et al. Thorax* 2000; **55**: 789–794.

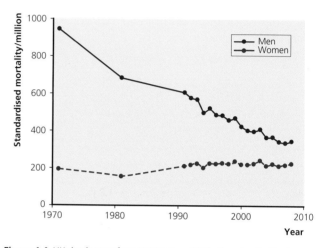

Figure 1.4 UK death rates from COPD since 1971. Age-standardised mortality rates per million: based on the European Standard Population. Figure derived with data from Death registrations, selected data tables, England and Wales 2008. Office for National Statistics, London. http://www.statistics.gov.uk/downloads/theme_health/DR2008/DR_08.pdf. (Accessed 12/09).

indices. This is because COPD is underdiagnosed due to failure to recognise the significance of symptoms and relatively late presentation of disease (Figure 1.1). Estimates of the prevalence of spirometric-defined COPD using UK criteria are less than the estimates based on European and US criteria (Chapter 4).

In the United Kingdom, a national study reported that 10% of males and 11% of females aged 16–65 years had an abnormally low forced expiratory volume in 1 second (FEV_1). Similarly, in Manchester, non-reversible airflow obstruction was present in 11% of subjects aged >45 years, of whom 65% had not been diagnosed with COPD. In Salzburg, Austria, doctor-confirmed COPD was reported by 5.6% of adults aged ≥40 years in a population survey; however, on evaluation using spirometric indices, 10.7% fulfilled UK criteria and 26.1% fulfilled European/US criteria. In the United States, the reported prevalence of airflow obstruction with an FEV_1 < 80% predicted was 6.8%, with 1.5% of the population having an FEV_1 < 50% and 0.5% of the population having more severe airflow obstruction (FEV_1 < 35% predicted). As in the United Kingdom, around 60% of subjects with airflow obstruction had not been formally diagnosed with COPD.

In England and Wales, it has been estimated that there are about 900,000 patients with diagnosed COPD. However, after allowing for underdiagnosis, the true number of individuals is likely to be about 1.5 million, although a figure as high as 3.7 million has been suggested. The mean age of diagnosis in the United Kingdom is around 67 years, and the prevalence of COPD increases with age (Figure 1.2). It is also more common in males and is associated with socio-economic deprivation. In the United Kingdom, the

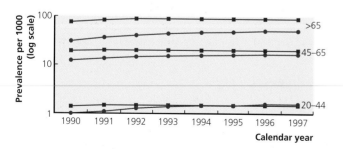

Figure 1.2 Prevalence (per 1000) of diagnosed COPD in UK men (■) and women (●) grouped by age, between 1990 and 1997. Reproduced with permission from Soriano JB, Maier WC, Egger P, *et al. Thorax* 2000; **55**: 789–794.

prevalence of COPD in females is increasing (Figures 1.3 and 1.4). For example, it was considered to be 0.8% in 1990 and had risen to 1.4% in 1997. In males, the prevalence appears to have plateaued since the mid-1990s. Similar trends have been reported in the United States. These time trends in prevalence probably reflect the gender differences in cigarette smoking since the 1970s.

Mortality

COPD is the fourth leading cause of death in the United States and Europe. Globally, COPD was ranked the sixth most common cause of death in 1990; however, with increases in life expectancy and cigarette smoking, particularly in developing countries, it is expected that COPD will be the third leading cause of death worldwide by 2020. In the United Kingdom in 2008, there were approximately 25,000 deaths due to COPD; 13,000 of these deaths were in males and 12,000 in females. These figures suggest that COPD underlies 4.9% of all deaths (5.4% of male deaths and 4.4% of female deaths) in the United Kingdom.

In the United Kingdom, over the last 30 years, mortality rates due to COPD have fallen in males and risen in females. However, it seems likely that in the near future, there will be no gender

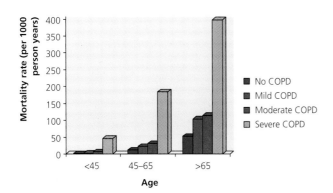

Figure 1.5 UK deaths from COPD (per 1000 person years) by age and severity of COPD. Figure derived with data from Soriano JB, Maier WC, Egger P, *et al*. Recent trends in physician diagnosed COPD in women and men in the UK. *Thorax* 2000; **55**: 789–794.

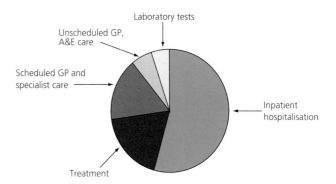

Figure 1.6 An analysis of the direct costs of COPD to the National Health Service. A&E, accident and emergency; GP, general practitioner. Figure derived with data from Britton M. The burden of COPD in the UK: results from the Confronting COPD survey. *Respiratory Medicine* 2003; **97**(suppl C): S71–S79.

difference. In the United States, the most recent data between 2000 and 2005 suggest that 5% of deaths are a consequence of COPD. Although overall, the age-standardised mortality rate was stable at about 64 deaths per 100,000, the death rate in males fell from 83.8/100,000 in 2000 to 77.3/100,000 in 2005 and increased in females from 54.4/100,000 to 56.0/100,000.

Mortality rates increase with age, disease severity and socio-economic disadvantage (Figure 1.5). On average, in the United Kingdom, COPD reduces life expectancy by 1.8 years (76.5 vs 78.3 years for controls); mild disease reduces life expectancy by 1.1 years, moderate disease by 1.7 years and severe disease by 4.1 years.

Morbidity and economic impact

The morbidity and economic costs associated with COPD are very high, generally unrecognised and more than twice that associated with asthma. The impact on quality of life is particularly high in patients with frequent exacerbations, although even those with mild disease have an impaired quality of life.

In the United Kingdom, emergency hospital admissions for COPD have steadily increased as a percentage of all admissions from 0.5% in 1991 to 1% in 2000. In 2002/2003, there were 110,000 hospital admissions for an exacerbation of COPD in England with an average duration of stay of 11 days, accounting for 1.1 million bed days. At least 10% of emergency admissions to hospital are as a consequence of COPD and this proportion is even greater during the winter. Most admissions are in individuals over 65 years of age with advanced disease who are often admitted repeatedly and use a disproportionate amount of resource. Approximately 25% of patients diagnosed with COPD are admitted to hospital and 15% of all patients are admitted each year.

The impact in primary care is even greater, with 86% of care being provided exclusively in that setting. It has been estimated that a typical general practitioner's list will include 200 patients with COPD (even more in areas of social deprivation), although not all will be diagnosed. On average, patients with COPD make six to seven visits annually to their general practitioner. It has been estimated that each diagnosed patient costs the UK economy £1639 annually, equating to a national burden of £982 million. For each patient, annual direct costs to the National Health Service (NHS)

are £819, with 54% of this being due to hospital admissions and 19% due to drug treatment (Figure 1.6). COPD has further societal costs; about 40% of UK patients are below retirement age and the disease prevents about 25% from working and reduces the capacity to work in a further 10%. Annual indirect costs have been estimated at £820 per patient and encompass the costs of disability, absence from work, premature mortality and the time caregivers miss work. Within Europe, it has been estimated that in 2001 the overall cost of COPD to the economy was €38.7 billion; this comprised of €4.7 billion for ambulatory care, €2.7 billion for drugs, €2.9 billion for inpatient care and €28.4 billion for lost working days.

Risk factors

Smoking

In developed countries, cigarette smoking is clearly the single most important risk factor in the development of COPD, with studies consistently reporting dose–response associations. Cigarette smoking is also associated with increased probability of COPD diagnosis and death. Pipe and cigar smokers have significantly greater morbidity and mortality from COPD than non-smokers, although the risk is less than that with cigarettes. Approximately 50% of cigarette smokers develop airflow obstruction and 10–20% develop clinically significant COPD. Maternal smoking during and after pregnancy is associated with reduced infant, childhood and adult ventilatory function, days, weeks and years after birth, respectively. Most studies have demonstrated that the effects of antenatal environmental tobacco smoking exposure are greater in magnitude and independent of associations with post-natal exposure.

Other factors

In the last 5 years, an increasing number of risk factors other than smoking have been linked to the development of COPD, particularly in developing countries. These include indoor (biomass) and out-door air pollution, occupational exposures and early life factors such as intra-uterine growth retardation, poor nutrition, repeated lower respiratory tract infections and a history of pulmonary tuberculosis. Many of these risk factors are inter-related. For example, biomass

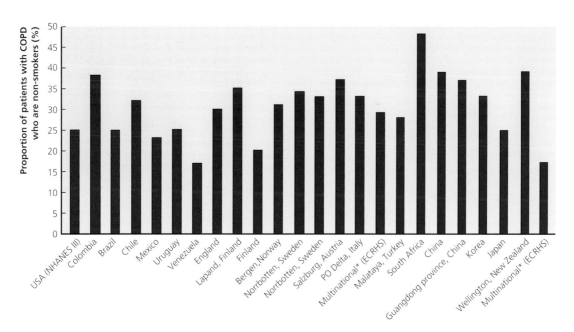

Figure 1.7 Proportion of patients with COPD who are non-smokers worldwide. ECRHS, European Community Respiratory Health Survey. Figure reproduced with permission from Salvi SS, Barnes PJ. Chronic obstructive pulmonary disease in non-smokers. *Lancet* 2009; **374**: 733–743. *Australia, Belgium, Denmark, France, Germany, Iceland, Ireland, Italy, Netherlands, New Zealand, Norway, Spain, Sweden, Switzerland, United Kingdom and United States.

smoke exposure is associated with intrauterine growth retardation and repeated early life lower respiratory tract infections. Accumulating evidence suggests that the prevalence of COPD worldwide in never smokers may be as high as 25–45% worldwide (Figure 1.7) with many risk factors and associations identified (Table 1.1).

Table 1.1 Non-smoking risk factors associated with the development of COPD.

Indoor air pollution
- Smoke from biomass fuel: plant residues (wood, charcoal, crops, twigs, dried grass) animal residues (dung)
- Smoke from coal

Occupational exposures
- Crop farming: grain dust, organic dust, inorganic dust
- Animal farming: organic dust, ammonia, hydrogen sulphide
- Dust exposures: coal mining, hard-rock mining, tunnelling, concrete manufacturing, construction, brick manufacturing, gold mining, iron and steel founding
- Chemical exposures: plastic, textile, rubber industries, leather manufacturing, manufacturing of food products
- Pollutant exposure: transportation and trucking, automotive repair

Treated pulmonary tuberculosis
Repeated childhood lower respiratory tract infections
Chronic asthma
Outdoor air pollution
- Particulate matter (<10 μm or <2.5 μm diameter)
- Nitrogen dioxide
- Carbon monoxide

Poor socio-economic status
Low educational attainment
Poor nutrition

Table reproduced with permission from Salvi SS, Barnes PJ. Chronic obstructive pulmonary disease in non-smokers. *Lancet* 2009; **374**: 733–743.

Air pollution

It has been demonstrated that urban air pollution may affect lung function development and consequently be a risk factor for COPD. Cross-sectional studies have demonstrated that higher levels of atmospheric air pollution are associated with cough, sputum production, breathlessness and reduced ventilatory function. Exposure to particulate and nitrogen dioxide air pollution has been associated with impaired ventilatory function in adults and reduced lung growth in children.

Worldwide, around 3 billion individuals are exposed to indoor air pollution from the use of biomass fuel (wood, charcoal, vegetable matter, animal dung) for cooking and heating; the smoke emitted contains pollutants such as carbon monoxide, nitrogen dioxide, sulphur dioxide, formaldehyde and particulate matter (Figure 1.8). It has been estimated that biomass smoke exposure underlies about 50% of diagnosed COPD in developing countries, with it being a particular problem in females and young children who are heavily exposed during cooking in poorly ventilated areas. Exposure to biomass smoke has been reported to increase the risk of COPD by two to threefold.

Occupation

Some occupational environments with intense prolonged exposure to irritating dusts, gases and fumes can cause COPD independently of cigarette smoking. However, smoking appears to enhance the effects of these occupational exposures. It has been estimated that about 15–20% of diagnosed cases are attributable to occupational hazards; in never smokers, this proportion increases to about 30%. Occupations that have been associated with a higher prevalence of COPD include coal mining, hard rock mining, tunnel working, concrete manufacturing, construction, farming, foundry

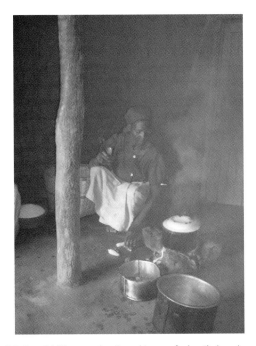

Figure 1.8 Over 2 billion people rely on biomass fuel as their main source of domestic energy; indoor air pollution associated with this, is an increasingly important cause of COPD in developing countries. Figure reproduced with permission from Dr Duncan Fullarton, Respiratory Infection Group, Liverpool School of Tropical Medicine, Liverpool, UK.

working, the manufacture of plastics, textiles, rubber, leather and food products, transportation and trucking. The increasing recognition that occupation can contribute to the development of COPD emphasises the importance of taking a full chronological occupational history.

Alpha-1-antitrypsin deficiency

The best documented genetic risk factor for airflow obstruction is α1-antitrypsin deficiency. However, this is a rare condition and is present in only 1–2% of patients with COPD. α1-Antitrypsin is a glycoprotein responsible for the majority of anti-protease activity in serum. The α1-antitrypsin gene is highly polymorphic, although some genotypes (usually ZZ) are associated with low serum levels (typically 10–20% of normal). Severe deficiency of α1-antitrypsin is associated with premature and accelerated development of COPD in smokers and non-smokers, although the rate of decline is greatly accelerated only in smokers. The α1-antitrypsin status of patients with severe COPD who are less than 40 years old should be determined since over 50% have α1-antitrypsin deficiency. The detection of affected individuals identifies family members who in turn require genetic counselling and patients who might be suitable for future potential treatment with α1-antitrypsin replacement.

Further reading

Britton M. The burden of COPD in the UK: results from the Confronting COPD survey. *Respiratory Medicine* 2003; **97**(suppl C): S71–S79.

Gibson PG, Simpson JL. The overlap syndrome of asthma and COPD: what are its features and how important is it? *Thorax* 2009; **64**: 728–735.

http://guidance.nice.org.uk/CG101/Guidance/pdf/English

Halbert RJ, Natoli JL, Gano A, Badamgarav E, Buist AS, Mannino DM. Global burden of COPD: systematic review and meta-analysis. *The European Respiratory Journal* 2006; **28**: 523–532.

Hu G, Zhou Y, Tian J *et al.* Risk of COPD from exposure to biomass smoke: a metaanalysis. *Chest* 2010; **138**: 20–31.

Lopez AD, Shibuya K, Rao C *et al.* Chronic obstructive pulmonary disease: current burden and future projections. *The European Respiratory Journal* 2006; **27**: 397–412.

Prescott E, Vestbo J. Socioeconomic status and chronic obstructive pulmonary disease. *Thorax* 1999; **54**: 737–741.

Pride NB, Soriano JB. Chronic obstructive pulmonary disease in the United Kingdom: trends in mortality, morbidity and smoking. *Current Opinion in Pulmonary Medicine* 2002; **8**: 95–101.

Salvi SS, Barnes PJ. Chronic obstructive pulmonary disease in non-smokers. *Lancet* 2009; **374**: 733–743.

Viegi G, Pistelli F, Sherrill DL, Maio S, Baldacci S, Carrozzi L. Definition, epidemiology and natural history of COPD. *The European Respiratory Journal* 2007; **30**: 993–1013.

CHAPTER 2

Pathology and Pathogenesis

William MacNee

MRC Centre for Inflammation Research, Queen's Medical Research Institute, University of Edinburgh, Edinburgh, UK

> **OVERVIEW**
>
> - The clinical sequelae of chronic obstructive pulmonary disease (COPD) results from pathological changes in the large airways (bronchitis), small airways (bronchiolitis) and alveolar space (emphysema)
> - Combinations of pathological changes occur to varying degrees in different individuals
> - Chronic inflammation – involving neutrophils, macrophages and T-lymphocytes – is found in the airways and alveolar space
> - Small airways inflammation (bronchiolitis) can lead eventually to scarring; this important pathological change is difficult to assess by conventional lung function tests, but is a major source of airway obstruction
> - In COPD, lungs show an amplified and persistent inflammatory response following exposure to particles and gases, particularly those found in cigarette smoke

Introduction

Chronic obstructive pulmonary disease (COPD) is characterised by chronic airflow limitation that is not fully reversible and an abnormal inflammatory response in the lungs. The latter represents the innate and adaptive immune responses to a lifetime of exposure to noxious particles, fumes and gases, particularly cigarette smoke. All cigarette smokers have inflammatory changes within their lungs, but those who develop COPD exhibit an enhanced or abnormal inflammatory response to inhaled toxic agents. This amplified or abnormal inflammatory response may result in mucous hypersecretion (chronic bronchitis), tissue destruction (emphysema), disruption of normal repair and defence mechanisms causing small airway inflammation (bronchiolitis) and fibrosis.

These pathological changes result in increased resistance to airflow in the small conducting airways and increased compliance and reduced elastic recoil of the lungs. This causes progressive airflow limitation and air trapping, which are the hallmark features of COPD. There is increasing understanding of the cell and the

molecular mechanisms that result in the pathological changes found and how these lead to physiological abnormalities and subsequent development of symptoms.

Pathology

The pathological changes in the lungs of patients with COPD are found in the proximal and peripheral airways, lung parenchyma and pulmonary vasculature. These changes are present to different extents in affected individuals (Box 2.1, Figures 2.1–2.3).

Box 2.1 **Pathological changes found in COPD**

Proximal airways (cartilaginous airways >2 mm in diameter)

- ↑ Macrophages and CD8 T-lymphocytes
- Few neutrophils and eosinophils (neutrophils increase with progressive disease)
- Submucosal bronchial gland enlargement and goblet cell metaplasia (results in excessive mucous production or chronic bronchitis)
- Cellular infiltrates (neutrophils and lymphocytes) of bronchial glands
- Airway epithelial squamous metaplasia, ciliary dysfunction, ↑ smooth muscle and connective tissue

Peripheral airways (non-cartilaginous airways <2 mm diameter)

- Bronchiolitis at an early stage
- ↑ Macrophages and T-lymphocytes (CD8 > CD4)
- Few neutrophils or eosinophils
- Pathological extension of goblet cells and squamous metaplasia into peripheral airways
- Luminal and inflammatory exudates
- ↑ B-lymphocytes, lymphoid follicles and fibroblasts
- Peribronchial fibrosis and airway narrowing with progressive disease

Lung parenchyma (respiratory bronchioles and alveoli)

- ↑ Macrophages and CD8 T-lymphocytes
- Alveolar wall destruction due to loss of epithelial and endothelial cells

---

ABC of COPD, 2nd edition.

Edited by Graeme P. Currie. © 2011 Blackwell Publishing Ltd.

- Development of emphysema (abnormal enlargement of airspaces distal to terminal bronchioles)
- Microscopic emphysematous changes:
  - centrilobular (dilatation and destruction of respiratory bronchioles – commonly found in smokers and predominantly in upper zones)
  - panacinar (destruction of the whole acinus – commonly found in α-1-antitrypsin deficiency and more common in lower zones)
- Macroscopic emphysematous changes:
  - microscopic changes progress to bullae formation (defined as an emphysematous airspace >1 cm in diameter)

Pulmonary vasculature

- ↑ Macrophages and T-lymphocytes
- Early changes:
  - intimal thickening
  - endothelial dysfunction
- Late changes:
  - ↑ vascular smooth muscle
  - collagen deposition
  - destruction of capillary bed
  - development of pulmonary hypertension and cor pulmonale

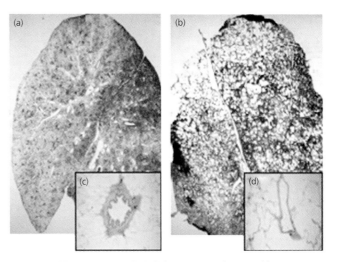

Figure 2.2 (a) Paper-mounted whole lung section of a normal lung; (b) paper-mounted whole lung section from a lung with severe central lobular emphysema. Note that the central lobular form is more extensive in the upper regions of the lung; (c) histological section of a normal small airway and surrounding alveoli connecting with attached alveolar walls; (d) histological section showing emphysema with enlarged alveolar spaces, loss of alveolar walls and alveolar attachments and collapsed airway.

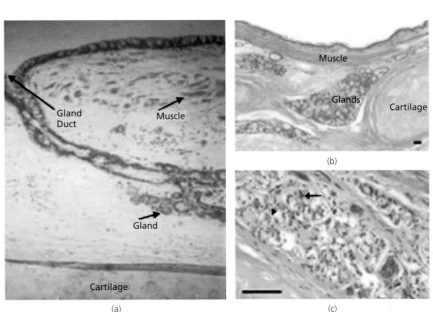

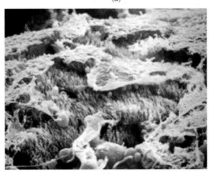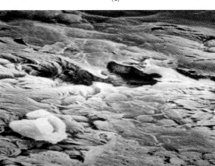

Figure 2.1 (a) A central bronchus from a cigarette smoker with normal lung function. Very small amounts of muscle and small epithelial glands are shown. (b) Bronchial wall from a patient with chronic bronchitis showing a thick bundle of muscle and enlarged glands. (c) A higher magnification of the enlarged glands from (b) showing chronic inflammation involving polymorphonuclear (arrow head) and mononuclear cells, including plasma cells (arrow). Printed with kind permission from JC Hogg and S Green. (d) Scanning electron micrograph of airway from a normal individual showing flakes of mucus overlying the cilia. (e) Scanning electron micrograph of a bronchial wall in a patient with chronic bronchitis. Cilia are covered with a blanket of mucus.

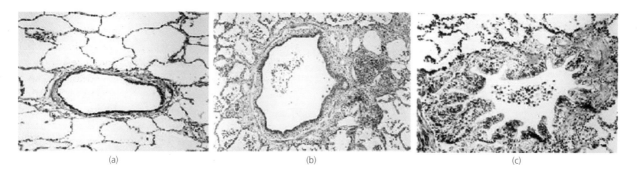

Figure 2.3 Histological sections of peripheral airways. (a) Section from a cigarette smoker with normal lung function showing a nearly normal airway with small numbers of inflammatory cells. (b) Section from a patient with small airway disease showing inflammatory exudate in the wall and lumen of the airway. (c) Section showing more advanced small airway disease, with reduced lumen causing structural reorganisation of the airway wall, increased smooth muscle and deposition of peribronchial connective tissue. Images produced with kind permission of Professor James C Hogg, University of British Columbia, Canada.

Pathogenesis

Inflammation is present in the lungs – particularly in the small airways – of all smokers. This normal protective response to inhaled toxins is amplified in COPD and leads to tissue destruction, impairment of defence mechanisms that limit such destruction and disruption of repair mechanisms. In general, the inflammatory and structural changes in the airways increase with disease severity and persist even after smoking cessation. A number of mechanisms are involved in intensifying lung inflammation, which results in the pathological changes in COPD (Figure 2.4).

Innate and adaptive immune inflammatory responses

The innate inflammatory immune system provides primary protection against the continuing insult of inhalation of toxic gases and particles. The first line of defence consists of the mucociliary clearance apparatus and macrophages that clear foreign material from the lower respiratory tract; both of these are impaired in COPD.

The second line of defence of the innate immune system is exudation of plasma and circulating cells into both large and small conducting airways and alveoli. This process is controlled by an array of proinflammatory chemokines and cytokines (Box 2.2).

Inflammatory cells

COPD is characterised by increased neutrophils, macrophages, T-lymphocytes (CD8 > CD4) and dendritic cells in various parts of the lungs (Box 2.2). In general, the extent of inflammation is related to the degree of airflow obstruction. These inflammatory cells are capable of releasing a variety of cytokines and mediators which participate in the disease process. This inflammatory cell pattern is markedly different from that found in asthma.

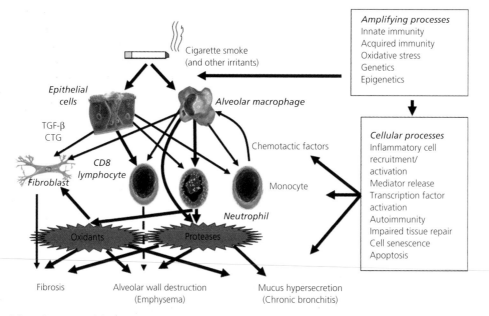

Figure 2.4 Overview of the pathogenesis of chronic obstructive pulmonary disease (COPD). Cigarette smoke activates macrophages in epithelial cells to produce chemotactic factors that recruit neutrophils and CD8 cells from the circulation. These cells release factors which activate fibroblasts, resulting in abnormal repair processes and bronchiolar fibrosis. Imbalance between proteases released from neutrophils and macrophages and antiproteases leads to alveolar wall destruction (emphysema). Proteases also cause the release of mucus. An increased oxidant burden resulting from smoke inhalation or release of oxidants from inflammatory leucocytes causes epithelial and other cells to release chemotactic factors, inactivates antiproteases and directly injures alveolar walls and causes mucus secretion. Several processes are involved in amplifying the inflammatory responses in COPD. TGF-β, transforming growth factor-β; CTG, connective tissue growth factor.

Inflammatory mediators

Many inflammatory mediators are increased in patients with COPD. These include

- leukotriene B$_4$ (LTB$_4$), a neutrophil and T-cell chemoattractant, which is produced by macrophages, neutrophils and epithelial cells;
- chemotactic factors such as CXC chemokines, interleukin-8 (IL-8) and growth-related oncogene-α produced by macrophages and epithelial cells; these attract cells from the circulation and amplify proinflammatory responses;
- proinflammatory cytokines such as tumour necrosis factor-α, IL-1β and IL-6;
- growth factors such as transforming growth factor-β (TGF-β), which may cause fibrosis in the airways either directly or through the release of another cytokine (connective tissue growth factor).

An adaptive immune response is also present in the lungs of patients with COPD, as shown by the presence of mature lymphoid follicles. These increase in number in the airways according to disease severity. Their presence has been attributed to the large antigen load associated with bacterial colonisation or frequent lower respiratory tract infections or possibly an autoimmune response. Dendritic cells are major antigen-presenting cells and are increased in the small airways, and provide a link between innate and adaptive immune responses.

Protease/antiprotease imbalance

Increased production (or activity) of proteases or inactivation (or reduced production) of antiproteases results in imbalance. Cigarette smoke and inflammation *per se* produce oxidative stress, which primes several inflammatory cells to release a combination of proteases and inactivate several antiproteases by oxidation. The major proteases involved in the pathogenesis of COPD are the serine proteases produced by neutrophils, cysteine proteases and matrix metalloproteases (MMPs) produced by macrophages. The major antiproteases involved in the pathogenesis of emphysema include α-1-antitrypsin, secretory leukoproteinase inhibitor and tissue inhibitors of MMP (Box 2.3).

Oxidative stress

The oxidative burden is increased in COPD. Sources of increased oxidants include cigarette smoke and reactive oxygen and nitrogen species released from inflammatory cells. This creates an imbalance in oxidants and antioxidants (oxidative stress). Many markers of oxidative stress are increased in stable COPD and are increased further during exacerbations. Oxidative stress can lead to inactivation of antiproteinases and stimulation of mucous production. It can also amplify inflammation by activating many intercellular pathways, including kinases (e.g. P38 mitogen-activated protein (MAP) kinase) enhancing transcription factor activation (e.g. nuclear factor-κB (NF-κB)) and epigenetic events (such as decreasing histone deacetylates) that lead to increased gene expression of proinflammatory mediators.

Emphysema is characterised by enlargement of the airspaces distal to the terminal bronchioles and is associated with destruction of alveolar walls but without fibrosis. Paradoxically, fibrosis may occur in the small airways in COPD. A number of mechanisms are involved in the pathogenesis of emphysema, including protease/antiprotease imbalance, oxidative stress, apoptosis and cell senescence (Box 2.4).

- Accelerated lung aging and cell senescence leading to failure of lung maintenance and repair
- Ineffective clearance of apoptotic cells (efferocytosis) by macrophages leading to decreased anti-inflammatory mechanisms
- Mitochondrial dysfunction with increased oxidative stress leading to increased cell apoptosis, for example through SIRT-1

MMP, Matrix metalloproteinase; VEGF, vascular endothelial growth factor; SIRT, sirtuin.

Pathophysiology

The pathogenic mechanisms described earlier result in the pathological changes found in COPD. These in turn cause physiological abnormalities such as mucous hypersecretion, ciliary dysfunction, airflow limitation and hyperinflation, gas exchange abnormalities, pulmonary hypertension and systemic effects.

Mucous hypersecretion and ciliary dysfunction

Mucous hypersecretion results in a chronic productive cough. This is characteristic of chronic bronchitis, but not necessarily associated with airflow limitation, while not all patients with COPD have symptomatic mucous hypersecretion. Mucous hypersecretion is due to an increased number of goblet cells and increased size of bronchial submucosal glands in response to chronic irritation caused by noxious particles and gases. Ciliary dysfunction is due to squamous metaplasia of epithelial cells and results in dysfunction of the mucociliary escalator and difficulty expectorating.

Airflow limitation and hyperinflation/ air trapping

Chronic airflow limitation is the physiological hallmark of COPD. The main site of airflow limitation occurs in the small conducting airways that are <2 mm in diameter. This is because of inflammation, narrowing (airway remodelling) and inflammatory exudates in the small airways. Other factors contributing to airflow limitation include loss of lung elastic recoil (due to destruction of alveolar walls) and destruction of alveolar support (from alveolar attachments).

The airway obstruction progressively traps air during expiration, resulting in hyperinflation of the lungs at rest and dynamic hyperinflation during exercise. Hyperinflation reduces the inspiratory capacity and, therefore, the functional residual capacity during exercise. These features result in the breathlessness and impaired exercise capacity typical of COPD.

Gas exchange abnormalities

Gas exchange abnormalities occur in advanced disease and are characterised by arterial hypoxaemia with or without hypercapnia. An abnormal distribution of ventilation/perfusion ratios – due to the

anatomic alterations described in COPD – is the main mechanism accounting for abnormal gas exchange. The extent of impairment of diffusing capacity for carbon monoxide is the best physiological correlate to the severity of emphysema.

Pulmonary hypertension

Pulmonary hypertension develops late in the course of COPD at the time of severe gas exchange abnormalities. Contributing factors include pulmonary arterial vasoconstriction (due to hypoxia), endothelial dysfunction, remodelling of the pulmonary arteries (smooth muscle hypertrophy and hyperplasia) and destruction of the pulmonary capillary bed.

The development of structural changes in the pulmonary arterioles results in persistent pulmonary hypertension and right ventricular hypertrophy/enlargement and dysfunction (Figure 2.5).

Systemic effects

COPD is associated with several extra-pulmonary effects (Box 2.5). The systemic inflammation and skeletal muscle wasting contribute to limiting the exercise capacity of patients and worsens prognosis, irrespective of the degree of airflow obstruction. There is an increased risk of cardiovascular disease in individuals with COPD and, if present, it is associated with a systemic inflammatory response and vascular dysfunction.

Box 2.5 **Systemic features of COPD**

- Cachexia
- Skeletal muscle wasting
- Increased risk of cardiovascular disease
- Normochromic normocytic anaemia
- Osteoporosis
- Depression
- Secondary polycythemia

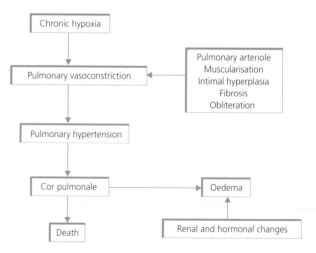

Figure 2.5 The development of pulmonary hypertension in chronic obstructive pulmonary disease (COPD).

Pathology, pathogenesis and pathophysiology of exacerbations

Exacerbations are often associated with increased neutrophilic inflammation in the airways, and in some mild exacerbations, the presence of increased numbers of eosinophils. Some exacerbations are infectious in origin (either bacterial or viral), while other potential mechanisms include air pollution and changes in ambient temperature. Viruses and bacteria may activate transcription factors such as NF-κB and the MAP kinases, leading to the release of inflammatory cytokines.

In mild exacerbations, the degree of airflow limitation is often unchanged or only slightly increased. Severe exacerbations are associated with worsening of pulmonary gas exchange due to increased ventilation/perfusion inequality and subsequent respiratory muscle fatigue. The worsening ventilation/perfusion relationship results from airway inflammation, oedema, mucous hypersecretion and bronchoconstriction. These reduce ventilation and cause hypoxic vasoconstriction of pulmonary arterioles, which in turn impairs perfusion.

Respiratory muscle fatigue and alveolar hypoventilation can contribute to hypoxaemia, hypercapnia, respiratory acidosis and lead to severe respiratory failure and death. Hypoxia and respiratory acidosis can induce pulmonary vasoconstriction, which increases the load on the right ventricle, and together with renal hormonal changes, can result in peripheral oedema.

Further reading

Chung KF, Adcock IM. Multifaceted mechanisms in COPD: inflammation, immunity, and tissue repair and destruction. *The European Respiratory Journal* 2008; **31**: 1334–1356.

Hogg JC. Lung structure and function in COPD. *The International Journal of Tuberculosis and Lung Disease* 2008; **12**: 467–479.

Hogg JC, Timens W. The pathology of chronic obstructive pulmonary disease. *Annual Review of Pathology* 2009; **4**: 435–459.

MacNee W. Pathogenesis of chronic pulmonary disease. *Clinics in Chest Medicine* 2007; **28**: 479–513.

Rodriguez-Roisin R, MacNee W. Pathophysiology of chronic obstructive pulmonary disease. *The European Respiratory Monograph* 2006; **11**: 177–200.

CHAPTER 3

Diagnosis

Graeme P. Currie and Mahendran Chetty

Aberdeen Royal Infirmary, Aberdeen, UK

OVERVIEW

- Chronic obstructive pulmonary disease (COPD) may be undiagnosed in its initial phase due to paucity of clinical features
- The diagnosis should be considered in any individual >35 years with breathlessness, chest tightness, wheeze, cough, sputum production and reduced exercise tolerance and who has a history of smoking (or other significant risk factor)
- Clinical examination may be normal in early disease
- All patients with suspected COPD need spirometry to confirm the diagnosis and grade the severity of airflow obstruction
- A chest X-ray and full blood count are mandatory at the time of diagnosis
- Other investigations such as detailed lung function tests, electrocardiogram, echocardiogram, chest computed tomography, pulse oximetry and arterial blood gases may be required in selected cases

---

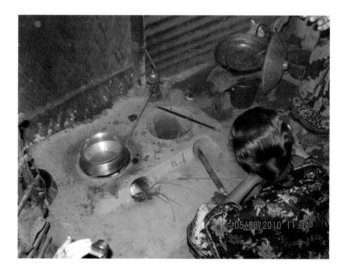

Figure 3.1 An example of an indoor fire used for cooking in a rural Indian village. Image reproduced with permission from Dr David Bellamy, retired Bournemouth General Practitioner.

As with most medical conditions, a thorough history should be taken and examination performed before embarking on investigations in a patient with possible or suspected chronic obstructive pulmonary disease (COPD). The diagnosis should be considered in individuals over 35 years of age with any relevant respiratory symptom and history of smoking (or other significant risk factor, e.g. exposure to indoor biomass fuels in developing countries) (Figure 3.1). The presence of airflow obstruction and severity of COPD are confirmed by spirometry; this remains the gold standard diagnostic test (Chapter 4).

Clinical features

Typical presenting symptoms

COPD may occur in any current or former smoker over the age of 35 years who complains of breathlessness, chest tightness, wheeze, chronic cough, sputum production, frequent winter chest infections or impaired exercise tolerance. The condition may also be present in the absence of troublesome respiratory symptoms, especially in those with a sedentary lifestyle or limited mobility.

Breathlessness may initially be noticed only during exertion, which later becomes progressive and persistent. It is useful to determine how breathlessness affects daily living activities such as walking on the flat (and walking distance), walking up inclines, climbing flights of stairs, carrying bags, walking to the shops, washing and dressing, doing light housework and hobbies. The impact of breathlessness on an individual's day-to-day life can be objectively assessed by the Medical Research Council (MRC) dyspnoea scale (Table 3.1). Chest tightness and wheeze (the high-pitched noise

Table 3.1 MRC breathlessness scale.

Grade	Degree of breathlessness related to activities
1	Not troubled by breathlessness except on strenuous exercise
2	Short of breath when hurrying or walking up a slight hill
3	Walks slower than contemporaries on the level because of breathlessness, or has to stop for breath when walking at own pace
4	Stops for breath after about 100 m or after a few minutes on the level
5	Too breathless to leave the house, or breathless when dressing or undressing

MRC, Medical Research Council.

ABC of COPD, 2nd edition.
Edited by Graeme P. Currie. © 2011 Blackwell Publishing Ltd.

Table 3.2 Causes of a chronic (lasting >8 weeks) cough.

Airway disorders	Parenchymal disease	Pleural disease	Others
COPD	Lung cancer	Pleural effusion	Gastro-oesophageal reflux disease
Asthma	Interstitial lung disease	Mesothelioma	Upper airway cough syndrome
Bronchiectasis including cystic fibrosis	Chronic lung infections (TB or fungal infections)		Angiotensin-converting enzyme inhibitor use
Smokers cough/ chronic bronchitis			Exposure to irritant dusts/chemicals/ fumes/particulate matter
Postviral hyperreactivity			

COPD, chronic obstructive pulmonary disease; TB, tuberculosis.

produced by air travelling through an abnormally narrowed smaller airway) may only be experienced during exertion or an exacerbation. Breathlessness, chest tightness and wheeze overnight are more suggestive of asthma. Chronic cough (defined as lasting >8 weeks) may be the presenting symptom in many other respiratory disorders (Table 3.2), and in COPD, is usually associated with sputum production. In healthy individuals, around 100 ml of sputum is produced daily, which is transported up the airway and swallowed; expectoration of excessive amounts of sputum is usually abnormal. In COPD, excessive amounts of sputum are often expectorated in the mornings and it is usually clear (mucoid), although it may also be light green because of nocturnal stagnation of neutrophils. During an exacerbation, sputum may be a darker green because of dead neutrophils. The initial presenting feature of COPD may also be with repeated lower respiratory tract infections, especially during winter months.

Other features in the history

As part of the overall assessment of COPD, it is essential to find out about symptoms of anxiety and depression, other medical conditions, current medication, frequency of exacerbations (and number of courses of steroids and antibiotics in the preceding year), previous hospital admissions, exercise limitation, occupational and environmental exposure to dust, chemicals and fumes, exposure to biomass fuel, previous chest problems (chronic asthma or tuberculosis), number of days missed from work and financial impact and the extent of social and family support. There is increasing evidence that COPD causes systemic effects, with anorexia and weight loss being relatively common and under-recognised problems in advanced COPD.

It is also important to determine when a patient started smoking, when he/she stopped smoking, the number of cigarettes smoked each day and the current smoking status. Patients should be asked about willingness to quit smoking and considered for referral to smoking cessation services. The number of smoking pack years can be calculated as follows:

- A one pack year is defined as 20 cigarettes (one pack) smoked per day for 1 year.

- Number of pack years = (number of cigarettes smoked per day × number of years smoked)/20.
- For example, a patient who has smoked 15 cigarettes per day for 40 years has a $(15 \times 40)/20 = 30$ pack year smoking history.

Signs

Signs of respiratory disease tend to appear as COPD progresses. Physical examination may therefore be normal, or reveal only prolongation of the expiratory phase of respiration or an elevated respiratory rate at rest in mild disease. In COPD, wheeze is usually heard during expiration (as airways normally dilate during inspiration and narrow in during expiration) and may occur only during exercise, in the morning (reflecting pooling of secretions blocking off smaller airways), or during an exacerbation. Late course inspiratory crackles are occasionally found in COPD, especially when excessive lower airway secretions are present.

As the disease progresses, examination may reveal a hyperinflated chest, increased anteroposterior diameter of the chest wall, intercostal indrawing, diminished breath sounds, wheezing at rest and faint heart sounds (due to hyperinflated lungs). Cyanosis (blue discolouration of the skin, lips and mucous membranes (Figure 3.2)), pursed lip breathing and use of accessory muscles (sternocleidomastoids, platysma and pectoral muscles) are features of advanced disease.

Cor pulmonale is present when right ventricular hypertrophy and pulmonary hypertension occurs as a consequence of any chronic lung disorder. Some patients with severe COPD may therefore demonstrate signs consistent with cor pulmonale (raised jugular venous pressure, loud P2 due to pulmonary hypertension, tricuspid regurgitation, pitting peripheral oedema (Figure 3.3) and hepatomegaly) and its presence usually indicates a poor prognosis. It may occur alongside features of CO_2 retention (warm peripheries, peripheral vasodilation and bounding pulse). Finger clubbing is *not* found in COPD and its presence should prompt thorough evaluation to exclude a cause such as lung cancer, bronchiectasis or idiopathic pulmonary fibrosis (Figure 3.4). Tar staining of the nails and fingers is commonly found in current or previous heavy cigarette smokers with COPD (Figure 3.5).

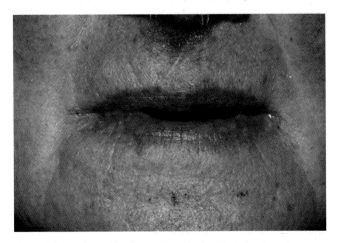

Figure 3.2 A patient with advanced hypoxic chronic obstructive pulmonary disease with central cyanosis.

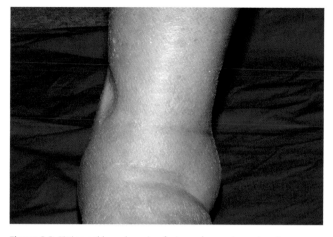

Figure 3.3 Pitting ankle oedema is a feature of cor pulmonale; other causes or contributory factors such as oral corticosteroids, calcium antagonists, excessive intravenous fluid administration, hypoalbumenaemia or dependant oedema should be considered.

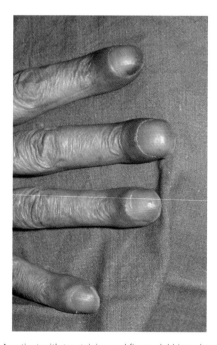

Figure 3.4 A patient with tar staining and finger clubbing; chronic obstructive pulmonary disease and non-small cell lung cancer were both diagnosed in this patient.

Skeletal muscle wasting and cachexia may occur in advanced disease, while some patients may also be overweight. The body mass index (BMI; weight/height^2) should be calculated during the initial examination. The BODE index (**B**MI, **O**bstruction, **D**yspnoea and **E**xercise) is a grading system which predicts the risk of death from any cause and from respiratory causes among patients with COPD (Table 3.3). A BODE index of 0–2, 3–4, 5–6 and 7–10 is thought to be associated with a 52-month mortality rate of approximately 10, 30, 50 and 80% respectively.

Differential diagnosis

Particular attention should be made to other features in the history and examination, which may suggest an alternative or concomitant

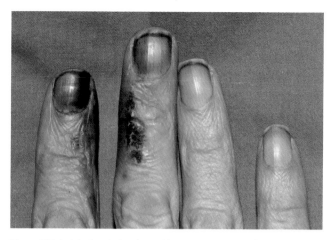

Figure 3.5 A right-handed patient with gross tar staining of the fingers due to chronic cigarette smoking.

Table 3.3 Calculation of the BODE index.

Parameter	Points				
	0	1	2	3	Score
BMI	≤21	>21			**0 or 1**
FEV$_1$ % predicted	≥65	50–64	36–49	≤35	**0, 1, 2 or 3**
Modified MRC scale	0–1	2	3	4	**0, 1, 2 or 3**
6-minute walk distance (metres)	≥350	250–349	150–249	≤149	**0, 1, 2 or 3**
					Total (out of 10)

The modified MRC scale uses the same clinical descriptors as the original MRC scale (1–5), although values are denoted as 0–4 in the calculation of the BODE index.
BODE, **B**MI, **O**bstruction, **D**yspnoea and **E**xercise; MRC, Medical Research Council.

disorder (Table 3.4). Since asthma tends to be the main differential diagnosis of COPD, a careful history should be taken in order to help distinguish between either disorder (Table 3.5). Symptoms such as haemoptysis, chest pain and weight loss require urgent referral to secondary care to rule out lung cancer or an alternative cardiorespiratory disorder.

Investigations

Lung function testing

Solitary peak expiratory flow (PEF) readings can significantly and seriously underestimate the extent of airflow obstruction, while serial monitoring of PEF is not generally useful in the diagnosis of COPD. Demonstration of airflow obstruction with spirometry is required to confirm the diagnosis. Spirometry is also useful in assessing severity of the disease and in following its progress plus response to treatment. The normal age-related decline in forced expiratory volume in 1 second (FEV$_1$) is around 20–40 ml/year and this increases to 40–80 ml/year in current smokers. More detailed lung function measurements such as lung volumes (total lung capacity and residual volume), gas transfer and 6-minute walk test can be performed if doubt exists in diagnosis or more thorough evaluation is required (such as during assessment for surgery or lung transplantation). Lung function testing in COPD is discussed in detail in Chapter 4.

Table 3.4 Conditions in the differential diagnosis of COPD.

Condition	Suggestive feature	Investigation
Asthma	Family history, atopy, non-smoker, young age, nocturnal symptoms	Trial of inhaled corticosteroids, reversibility testing if airflow obstruction present
Congestive cardiac failure	Orthopnoea, history of ischaemic heart disease, fine lung crackles	Chest X-ray, electrocardiogram, echocardiogram
Lung cancer	Haemoptysis, weight loss, hoarseness	Chest X-ray, bronchoscopy, CT
Bronchiectasis	Copious sputum production, frequent chest infections, childhood pneumonia, coarse lung crackles	Sputum microscopy, culture and sensitivity, high-resolution CT
Interstitial lung disease	Dry cough, history of connective tissue disease, use of drugs such as methotrexate, amiodarone, etc., fine lung crackles	Pulmonary function testing, chest X-ray, high-resolution CT, lung biopsy, autoantibodies
Opportunistic infection	Dry cough, risk factors for immunosuppression, fever	Chest X-ray, sputum microscopy, culture and sensitivity, induced sputum, bronchoalveolar lavage
Tuberculosis	Weight loss, haemoptysis, night sweats, risk factors for tuberculosis and immunosuppression	Chest X-ray, sputum microscopy, culture and sensitivity

COPD, chronic obstructive pulmonary disease, CT, computed tomography.

Table 3.5 Clinical differences between COPD and asthma.

	COPD	Asthma
Age	>35 years	Any age
Cough	Persistent and productive	Intermittent and non-productive
Smoking	Almost invariable	Possible
Breathlessness	Progressive and persistent	Intermittent and variable
Nocturnal symptoms	Uncommon unless in severe disease	Common
Family history	Uncommon unless family members also smoke	Common
Concomitant eczema or allergic rhinitis	Possible	Common

COPD, chronic obstructive pulmonary disease.

Imaging

All patients with suspected COPD should have a posteroanterior chest X-ray performed at diagnosis. This may be normal, although as the disease progresses, hyperinflation (flattened diaphragms, a narrowed heart, >6 anterior rib ends visible and 'squared off apices') and hyperlucency of lung fields may be evident (Figure 3.6). A chest X-ray also helps discount other causes of respiratory symptoms and identify complications related to COPD such as bullae formation and pulmonary arterial hypertension (enlarged central pulmonary arteries and peripheral arterial pruning). There is no direct link between extent of chest X-ray abnormality and degree of airflow obstruction. When there is doubt in diagnosis or a surgical procedure contemplated (such as lung volume reduction surgery or bullectomy), high-resolution computed tomographic (HRCT) imaging of the chest is required (Figure 3.7).

Other investigations

All patients should have a full blood count checked; this may show secondary polycythaemia, and excludes anaemia as a cause of chronic breathlessness. The discovery of a raised eosinophil count should raise the possibility of an alternative diagnosis such as asthma or eosinophilic pneumonia.

In patients with signs of cor pulmonale, an electrocardiogram may show changes of chronic right-sided heart strain (Figure 3.8). However, an echocardiogram is more sensitive in detecting tricuspid valve incompetence along with right atrial and ventricular hypertrophy and may also indirectly assess pulmonary artery pressure. Moreover, echocardiography is also a useful tool to determine whether left ventricular dysfunction is present, especially when

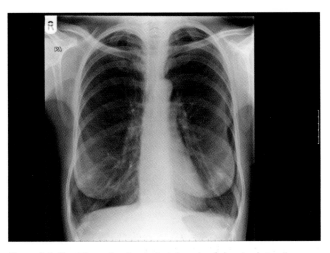

Figure 3.6 Chest X-ray showing typical changes of chronic obstructive pulmonary disease (>6 ends of anterior ribs visible, flat diaphragms and increased translucency of lung fields).

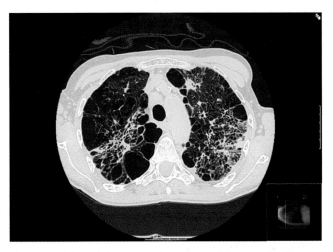

Figure 3.7 High-resolution computed tomogram of the chest showing widespread upper lobe emphysematous bullae in a patient with advanced COPD.

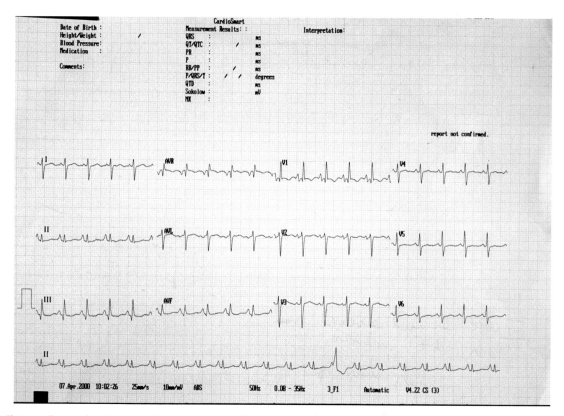

Figure 3.8 Electrocardiogram showing typical changes in a patient with cor pulmonale (p-pulmonale, right-axis deviation, partial right bundle branch block).

the spirometric impairment is disproportional to the extent of breathlessness. It is also important to be aware that ischaemic heart disease may be the sole or contributory cause of breathlessness (anginal equivalent) even in the absence of chest pain and investigations should be tailored accordingly. Indeed, dyspnoea due to causes other than COPD should be considered when the extent of physical limitation appears disproportionate to the degree of airflow obstruction.

Individuals with a family history of COPD, or when it presents at a young age, (especially when smoking pack years are negligible) should have α-1-antitrypsin levels checked. α-1-Antitrypsin deficiency is an autosomal codominant genetic disorder associated with the early development of airflow obstruction, panacinar emphysema and liver dysfunction. Necrotising panniculitis and Wegener's granulomatosis are infrequent complications. If α-1-antitrypsin deficiency is discovered, appropriate family screening and counselling, along with strict advice on smoking cessation, is warranted.

Assessment of pulse oximetry is useful in most patients, especially when more advanced disease ($FEV_1 < 50\%$ predicted) or polycythaemia is present, to detect the possibility of significant hypoxaemia. Patients with a resting oxygen saturation of <92% should have measurement of arterial blood gases, and where necessary and appropriate, be considered for assessment for long-term domiciliary or ambulatory oxygen.

Further reading

Celli BR, Cote CG, Marin JM *et al*. The body-mass index, airflow obstruction, dyspnea, and exercise capacity index in chronic obstructive pulmonary disease. *The New England Journal of Medicine* 2004; **350**: 1005–1012.

http://www.goldcopd.org

http://guidance.nice.org.uk/CG101/Guidance/pdf/English

Siafakas NM, Vermeire P, Pride NB *et al*. Optimal assessment and management of chronic obstructive pulmonary disease (COPD). A consensus statement of the European Respiratory Society (ERS). *The European Respiratory Journal* 1995; **8**: 1398–1420.

CHAPTER 4

Spirometry

David Bellamy

Bournemouth General Practitioner (retired), Bournemouth, UK

OVERVIEW

- Spirometry is the gold standard investigation in the diagnosis (and exclusion) of chronic obstructive pulmonary disease (COPD) and in assessing its severity
- In the presence of consistent symptoms, clinically significant COPD can be diagnosed when forced expiratory volume in 1 second/forced vital capacity (FEV_1/FVC) <0.7 *and* FEV_1 < 80% predicted
- Spirometry helps differentiate COPD from asthma and other respiratory conditions
- Spirometry readings – when performed correctly – are accurate, reliable and repeatable
- Approved educational courses for operators are essential to maintain a high-quality spirometry service

Introduction

While history and examination are essential in the diagnostic workup of suspected chronic obstructive pulmonary disease (COPD), demonstrating airflow obstruction is vital in confirming the diagnosis. Spirometry is recommended as being mandatory by all national guidelines and it should therefore be arranged in all individuals in whom the diagnosis of COPD is considered.

Spirometry was traditionally performed in hospital lung function laboratories and respiratory outpatient clinics. However, over the last 5 years – largely prompted by the widespread dissemination of national guidelines and the Quality Outcomes Framework system – there has been a major shift in spirometry being performed in primary care, with over 80% of practices now having this capability. Surveys of primary care use of spirometry have unfortunately raised major concerns regarding technical performance and quality and interpretation of results. Training in spirometry for general practitioners and nurses is highly variable and implies that there is need for attendance at properly accredited courses such as those run by the British Thoracic Society and Association for Respiratory Technology and Physiology.

ABC of COPD, 2nd edition.
Edited by Graeme P. Currie. © 2011 Blackwell Publishing Ltd.

What is spirometry?

Spirometry is a method of assessing lung function by measuring the volume of air that can be expelled from the lungs following maximal inspiration. The indices derived from this forced expiratory manoeuvre have become the most accurate, repeatable and reliable way of confirming the diagnosis of COPD. When these values are compared to predicted normal values, the presence (or absence) of COPD – and its severity – can be confirmed.

Why perform spirometry?

Spirometry is the best way of detecting the presence of airflow obstruction and making a definitive diagnosis of COPD. To make a diagnosis of COPD, the postbronchodilator forced expiratory volume in 1 second (FEV_1)/forced vital capacity (FVC) ratio needs to be <0.7 *and* FEV_1 < 80% of predicted. If the FEV_1 is ≥80% predicted of normal, a diagnosis of COPD should only be made in the presence of typical respiratory symptoms, for example breathlessness or cough. Spirometry can also help assess response to treatment and monitor disease progression. Demonstration of abnormal lung function results may help motivate individuals who smoke to quit. However, the FEV_1 in isolation is poorly linked to prognosis, quality of life and functional status.

An alternative diagnosis should be considered in older patients without typical symptoms of COPD where the FEV_1/FVC ratio is <0.7 and in younger patients with symptoms of COPD where the FEV_1/FVC ratio is ≥0.7.

Types of spirometer

Different types of spirometers exist and are used in differing clinical settings. Large bellows or rolling-seal spirometers are not portable and are used mainly in lung function laboratories. They require regular calibration, but provide very accurate measurements. Desktop spirometers are compact, portable and quick and easy to use. They usually have a real-time visual display and provide a paper printout. Some require calibration and others can be checked for accuracy with a 3-l syringe; any changes need to be made by the manufacturer. Generally, they require little maintenance other than cleaning. Desktop spirometers maintain accuracy over years and are ideal

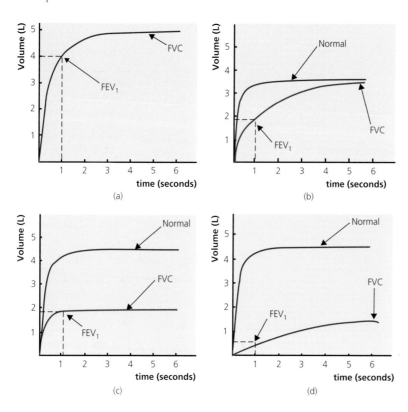

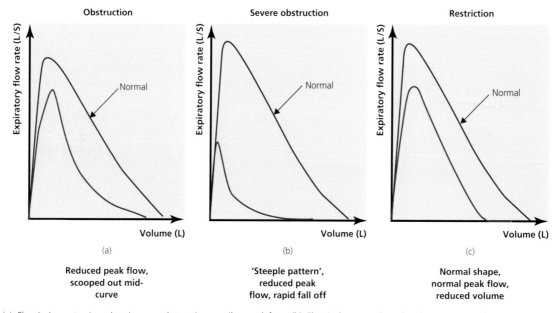

Figure 4.1 (a) Normal volume/time tracing. (b) Volume/time tracing showing an obstructive ventilatory defect; note the reduced forced expiratory volume in 1 second (FEV_1) and normal forced vital capacity (FVC). (c) Volume/time tracing showing a restrictive ventilatory defect; note the proportionally reduced FEV_1 and FVC. (d) Volume/time tracing showing a mixed obstructive and restrictive ventilatory defect; note that both the FEV_1 and FVC are disproportionally reduced.

Figure 4.2 (a) Flow/volume tracing showing an obstructive ventilatory defect. (b) Flow/volume tracing showing a severe obstructive ventilatory defect. (c) Flow/volume tracing showing a restrictive ventilatory defect.

for use in primary care. Small, inexpensive hand-held spirometers provide a numerical record of forced expiratory manoeuvres but not a printout. These devices are useful for simple screening and are still accurate for diagnosis if a desktop spirometer is unavailable.

Many spirometers provide two forms of traces. One is a plot of volume of air exhaled versus time (Figure 4.1a–d), while the other is a plot of flow versus volume of air exhaled. The latter is called a *flow/volume trace* and is helpful in identifying airflow obstruction (Figure 4.2a–c).

Spirometric indices

The standard manoeuvre is a maximal forced exhalation (with greatest effort possible) after a maximum deep inspiration (to total lung capacity). Several indices can be derived from this manoeuvre. These include the following:

- FVC – the total volume of air that can be forcibly exhaled in one breath.
- FEV_1 – the volume of air that can be exhaled in the first second of forced expiration.
- FEV_1/FVC – the ratio of FEV_1 to FVC (expressed as a decimal).

The FEV_1 and FVC are measured in litres and are also expressed as a percentage of the predicted values for that individual. Predicted values are calculated from normal individuals and vary with gender, height, age and ethnicity. The standard predicted values in most of Europe are those selected by the European Respiratory Society or the European Community Health and Respiratory Survey (ECHRS). Other predicted values may be used in different countries, although those most appropriate for the local population should be used.

The ratio of FEV_1/FVC is normally between 0.7 and 0.8. Values <0.7 indicate airflow obstruction, although in older adults, values between 0.65 and 0.7 may be normal. Using 0.7 as a cut off may therefore lead to overdiagnosis of COPD in the elderly. The FEV_1/FVC ratio is ≥ 0.7 in restrictive ventilatory defects.

Other measurements

- Forced expiratory volume in 6 seconds (FEV_6) – this is a more recently derived value, which measures the volume of air that can be forcibly exhaled in 6 seconds. It approximates the FVC, and in healthy individuals, the FEV_6 and FVC are identical. Using FEV_6 instead of FVC may be helpful in patients with more severe airflow obstruction who can take up to 15 seconds to fully exhale.
- Slow vital capacity (slow VC) – this parameter is obtained when the patient inhales to total lung capacity and exhales more slowly. In patients with more advanced airflow obstruction and dynamic compression, the slow VC may exceed the FVC by 0.5 l. International guidelines in the future may suggest that the FEV_1/slow VC is the preferred ratio by which to identify airflow obstruction.
- Forced mid-expiratory flow (FEF_{25-75}) – this is the flow of air forcibly exhaled between 25% and 75% of the FVC manoeuvre; this value may be reflective of airflow obstruction in smaller airways.

Interpretation and classification of spirograms

Interpretation of spirometry involves looking at the absolute values of FEV_1, FVC and FEV_1/FVC ratio, comparing them with predicted values and examining the shape of traces (Tables 4.1 and 4.2). Patients should complete three manoeuvres that are within 5% or 100 ml of each other; some electronic spirometers automatically provide this information.

The volume/time curve should rise rapidly and smoothly, and plateau within 3–4 seconds (Figure 4.1a). With increasing degrees of airflow obstruction, it takes longer to completely exhale (i.e.

Table 4.1 Features of normal, obstructive, restrictive and mixed obstructive/restrictive spirometry.

Pattern	FEV_1	FVC	FEV_1/FVC
Normal	$\geq$80% predicted	$\geq$80% predicted	0.7–0.8
Obstructive	<80% predicted	>80% predicted (or <80% predicted in advanced disease)	<0.7
Restrictive	<80% predicted	<80% predicted (FEV_1 and FVC are reduced proportionally)	$\geq$0.7
Mixed obstructive/ restrictive	<80% predicted	<80% predicted (FEV_1 is reduced to a greater extent than FVC)	<0.7

FEV_1, forced expiratory volume in 1 second; FVC, forced vital capacity.

Table 4.2 Causes of obstructive and restrictive spirometry.

Obstructive disorders	Restrictive disorders
COPD	Neuromuscular disorders
Symptomatic asthma	Interstitial lung disease
Bronchiectasis	Kyphoscoliosis
	Pleural effusion
	Morbid obesity
	Previous pneumonectomy

COPD, chronic obstructive pulmonary disease.

reach residual volume) – sometimes up to 15 seconds – and the upward slope of the spirogram is less steep (Figure 4.1b).

Bronchodilator reversibility testing

Spirometry before and after treatment with bronchodilators or corticosteroids (reversibility testing) is not necessary in suspected COPD, although doing so should be considered when asthma is thought likely or when the response to treatment is surprisingly good. However, asthma can usually be differentiated from COPD on account of the history, examination and baseline spirometry (which is usually normal outwith an exacerbation). However, recently updated NICE guidelines suggest that baseline postbronchodilator spirometry should ideally be performed at the time of diagnosis.

An improvement of >400 ml in FEV_1 following β_2-agonists or corticosteroids strongly suggests that asthma is the diagnosis. To check for reversibility, spirometry should be performed at baseline and 20 minutes after 400 µg of inhaled (or 2.5 mg of nebulised) salbutamol. Alternative options include spirometry before and after prednisolone 30 mg/day for 2 weeks or inhaled beclomethasone 400 µg/day for 6–8 weeks.

Severity of airflow obstruction in COPD

The severity of airflow obstruction in COPD can be categorised according to the degree of impairment of the FEV_1% predicted. However, there is no international agreement in terms of classification of severity; similarities and differences are shown in Table 4.3.

Table 4.3 Classification of airflow obstruction in COPD according to different guidelines; values shown are all FEV_1% predicted and in all categories post-bronchodilator $FEV_1/FVC < 0.7$.

Severity of airflow obstruction	NICE 2010	ATS/ERS 2004	GOLD 2008
Mild	$FEV_1 \geq 80\%$ (with compatible symptoms)	$FEV_1 \geq 80\%$	$FEV_1 \geq 80\%$
Moderate	FEV_1 50–79%	FEV_1 50–79%	FEV_1 50–79%
Severe	FEV_1 30–49%	FEV_1 30–49%	FEV_1 30–49%
Very severe	$FEV_1 < 30\%$ (or when $< 50\%$ with respiratory failure)	$FEV_1 < 30\%$	$FEV_1 < 30\%$ (or $FEV_1 < 50\%$ with respiratory failure)

NICE, National Institute for Clinical Excellence; ATS/ERS, American Thoracic Society/European Respiratory Society; GOLD, Global Initiative for Chronic Obstructive Lung Disease.

Flow/volume measurement

Most electronic spirometers measure airflow, which allows the flow rate against the volume to be plotted (flow/volume curve) (Figure 4.2a–c). Flow/volume interpretation is a helpful addition to interpreting lung function results and provides a quick and simple check as to whether airflow obstruction is present. It may also identify early stages of airflow obstruction and provide additional help when faced with the interpretation of a mixed pattern of obstruction and restriction.

- A normal trace will have a rapid rise to maximal expiratory flow followed by an almost linear uniform decline in flow until all the air is exhaled.
- In airflow obstruction, a concave dip in the second part of the curve is found, which becomes more marked with increasing obstruction (Figure 4.2a).
- In more severe COPD where loss of airway elasticity causes airways to collapse during forced exhalation, a characteristic sudden fall in flow occurs after maximal expiratory flow is reached – the so-called *steeple curve* (Figure 4.2b).
- In restrictive ventilatory defects, the shape of the flow–volume curve is normal but a reduction in lung volume – which moves the FVC point to the left compared with the predicted curve – occurs (Figure 4.2c).

How to perform spirometry

Spirometry should be undertaken when the patient is clinically stable. Ideally, short-acting bronchodilators should be withheld for the previous 6 hours, long-acting bronchodilators for 12 hours and sustained release theophylline for 24 hours. When performing spirometry for the first time, most patients (once comfortably seated) need clear, concise and unhurried instruction by a skilled and experienced operator. The following practical points need to be followed:

- Record the patient's age, height and gender and enter into the spirometer or computer.
- Note ethnicity and add correction factor if required.

- Document when bronchodilator was last used.
- Attach a clean, disposable, one-way mouthpiece to the spirometer.
- The use of a nose clip is optional.
- Ask patients to breathe in fully until the 'lungs feel full'.
- Ask patients to hold their breath long enough to seal their lips tightly around the mouthpiece.
- Ask patients to 'blast' air out as forcibly and as fast as possible until there is no more air left to expel; the operator should encourage the patient to keep blowing during this phase.
- Observe the patient carefully during the manoeuvre.
- Check that an adequate trace has been achieved; with electronic spirometers, leak of a small volume of air into the mouthpiece while sealing the lips may register as an attempt.
- Ask the patient to repeat the manoeuvre at least 3 times until three acceptable and reproducible traces are obtained (with a maximum of eight efforts).
- The best two traces should be within 100 ml or 5% of each other.
- Record the highest FEV_1 and FVC obtained.

Contraindications to spirometry

There are few absolute contraindications to performing spirometry, but it should probably not be pursued in any of the following circumstances:

- Recent (in the last month) myocardial infarct, uncontrolled hypertension or stroke
- Moderate or large volume haemoptysis of unknown origin
- Known or suspected pneumonia and tuberculosis
- Recent or current pneumothorax
- Recent thoracic, abdominal or eye surgery

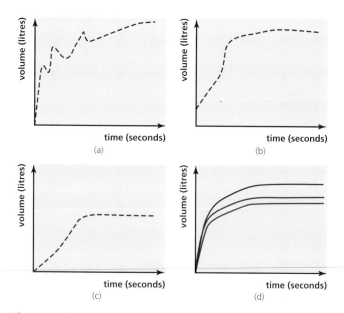

Figure 4.3 (a) Poor spirometry trace due to coughing. (b) Poor spirometry trace due to inconsistent effort. (c) Poor spirometry trace due to a 'slow' start. (d) Poor spirometry traces due to several suboptimal efforts (or patient becoming tired).

Accuracy and quality of traces

The most common cause for a poor-quality trace (Figure 4.3a–d) is suboptimal patient performance (sometimes due to inadequate explanation by the operator). It is therefore important to observe the patient throughout the manoeuvre and provide advice on how to improve technique. Common problems and pitfalls include the following:

- Inadequate or incomplete inhalation (to total lung capacity)
- Lack of 'blast effort' during exhalation
- Incomplete emptying of lungs to residual volume (common in COPD where it can take up to 15 seconds)
- An additional breath inwards during the expiratory manoeuvre
- Lips not tight around the mouthpiece (leaks underestimate FEV_1 and FVC)
- A slow start to the expiratory manoeuvre (doing so underestimates FEV_1)
- Exhaling to some extent through the nose
- Coughing
- Poor posture (e.g. leaning excessively forwards or backwards)

Equipment maintenance and calibration

To provide accurate and repeatable results, spirometers must be regularly cleaned and maintained according to the manufacturer's instructions. Calibration should be performed on a regular basis and the frequency of doing so depends on the individual spirometer.

Infection control

Precautions are necessary to minimise any cross-infection between patients via the spirometer and its mouthpiece. The use of barrier filters and disposable mouthpieces significantly reduces the risk of infection and helps protect equipment from exhaled secretions. A new filter must be used for each patient.

Training

Training is a key issue in successfully performing spirometry and interpreting results. Those involved in doing so should attend an accredited course to gain a full basic training. Regular updates of ability and knowledge on interpretation of results are also desirable.

Further reading

Levy M, Quanjer PH, Booker R, Cooper BG, Holmes S, Small I. Diagnostic spirometry in primary care. Proposed standards for general practice compliant with American Thoracic Society and European Respiratory Society recommendations. *Primary Care Respiratory Journal* 2009; **18**: 130–147.

Spirometry in Practice: A Practical Guide to Using Spirometry in Primary Care, 2nd edn. (www.brit-thoracic.org.uk/Portals/0/Clinical%20Information/COPD/COPD%20Consortium/spirometry_in_practice051.pdf).

CHAPTER 5

Smoking Cessation

John Britton

UK Centre for Tobacco Control Studies, University of Nottingham, Nottingham, UK *and*
City Hospital, Nottingham, UK

OVERVIEW

- Smoking is the biggest avoidable cause of chronic obstructive pulmonary disease (COPD) in developed countries
- Smoking cessation is the only intervention which has a sustained and significant effect on the natural history of COPD
- Preventing smoking uptake, and promoting smoking cessation, is the most effective means of preventing COPD and reducing rates of progression
- Preventing uptake of smoking involves 'denormalising' smoking in society; this means that schoolchildren should not develop the belief that smoking is a normal or even desirable adult behaviour
- Healthcare workers should encourage all individuals to quit smoking at every available opportunity and support those who are willing to try
- Smoking cessation is much more likely to be successful if a combination of behavioural support with nicotine replacement therapy, varenicline or bupropion is used

---

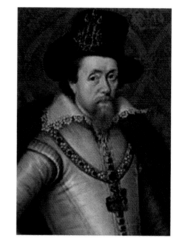

Figure 5.1 King James I of England.

Effects of cigarette smoking

Apart from being one of the most common and important causes of chronic obstructive pulmonary disease (COPD), cigarette smoking causes a range of other chronic diseases and cancers affecting almost every bodily system (Table 5.1). Cigarette smoking results in over 100 000 deaths each year in the United Kingdom, and most of these are due to COPD, lung cancer or ischaemic heart disease. Some diseases, including sarcoidosis, extrinsic allergic alveolitis, Parkinson's disease and ulcerative colitis are less common in smokers.

Primary prevention of COPD

Preventing smoking will do more to prevent COPD than any other measure. However, as long as cigarette smoking remains a

Smoking was introduced into the United Kingdom in the late 16th century. Shortly afterwards, the son of Mary Queen of Scots, King James I of England (Figure 5.1), was the first monarch to implement a tax on tobacco use. He also published his famous *Counterblaste to tobacco* in 1604 where he reflected on his dislike of the 'precious stink' and observed that:

Smoking is a custom loathsome to the eye, hateful to the nose, harmful to the brain, dangerous to the lungs, and in the black, stinking fume thereof nearest resembling the horrible Stygian smoke of the pit that is bottomless.

Cigarette smoking delivers nicotine – a powerfully addictive drug – quickly and in high doses directly to the brain. Addiction to nicotine is usually established through experimentation with cigarettes during adolescence and commonly results in sustained or even lifelong smoking. However, nicotine itself does not cause major health problems in most users, as it is tar that accompanies nicotine that causes most of the harm.

Table 5.1 Effects of cigarette smoking, other than causing COPD.

Cancers	Chronic diseases	Miscellaneous
Lung	Ischaemic heart disease	Respiratory tract infections
Oropharyngeal	Hypertension	Complications of diabetes
Oesophagus	Cerebrovascular disease	Infertility and impotence
Bladder	Peripheral vascular disease	Premature aging
Stomach	Macular degeneration	Increased skin wrinkling
Pancreatic	Osteoporosis	Persistent symptoms of asthma

COPD, chronic obstructive pulmonary disease.

ABC of COPD, 2nd edition.
Edited by Graeme P. Currie. © 2011 Blackwell Publishing Ltd.

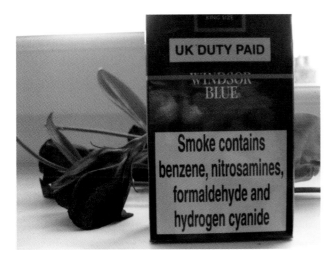

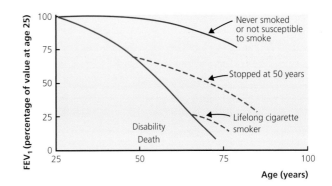

Figure 5.3 Beneficial effects of smoking cessation occur at any age. FEV_1, forced expiratory volume in 1 second. Figure reproduced with permission from Hogg JC. Pathophysiology of airflow limitation in chronic obstructive pulmonary disease. *Lancet* 2004; **364**: 709–721.

Figure 5.2 Warnings found on cigarette boxes are useful ways in which to remind individuals of the dangers of smoking.

normal and acceptable behaviour in adults, children and adolescents will continue to experiment with and become addicted to smoking. Measures to reduce access to cigarettes by young people will help prevent some from starting to smoke, but the more important preventive strategies are general population measures that 'denormalise' smoking in society. Examples include

- comprehensive bans on advertising and promotion, including point of sale displays;
- sustained increases in real price;
- policing of illegal sources of less-expensive cigarettes;
- comprehensive smoke-free policies at work and in public places;
- health warnings on cigarette packs (Figure 5.2);
- sustained health promotion campaigns.

Smoking cessation

Smoking cessation is the most effective means of preventing COPD or reducing the rate of progression in established disease. Smoking cessation reduces the rate of decline in lung function in individuals with COPD to that of a non-smoker (Figure 5.3). Individuals with COPD who quit smoking also experience a substantial improvement in overall health, functional status and survival, in addition to a reduced incidence of many forms of cancer and cardiovascular disease. Thus, it is important to emphasise to all patients with COPD that it is never too late to stop smoking.

Highly successful and cost-effective smoking cessation interventions have been available for many years. These include generic population measures to encourage smoking cessation (and discourage uptake of smoking), in addition to individual interventions involving behavioural support and pharmacotherapy.

Helping patients with COPD stop smoking

Behavioural support

All health professionals should give brief advice to encourage all smokers to quit at every available opportunity (Box 5.1). Advice should be offered in an encouraging, non-judgemental

and empathetic manner, and supported where possible by written information (Figure 5.4). Some examples of approaches to take in discussing smoking are listed below; behavioural strategies to encourage are listed in Box 5.2.

- Explain that stopping smoking is not easy and that several attempts may be required to achieve long-term success.
- Find out if the individual is motivated to stop, and if so, support a quit attempt as soon as possible. If not motivated, explore reasons for not quitting and encourage the smoker to consider doing so in the future.
- Introduce the notion that cigarette is a killer and should not be regarded as the 'comforting friend' in times of anxiety and stress.
- Explain that cigarette smoking feels pleasurable or relaxing, primarily because it relieves nicotine withdrawal symptoms – remind individuals of their first experience of cigarette smoking and ask if it was pleasant.
- List the number of harmful chemicals and carcinogens (such as benzene and arsenic) that are found in cigarettes and all the other diseases caused by cigarette smoking.

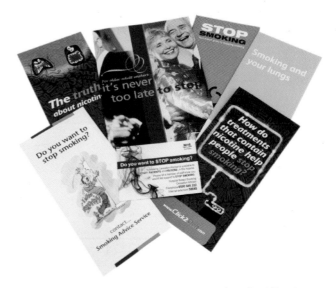

Figure 5.4 Verbal and written smoking cessation advice should be given to all current smokers.

- Stress the importance of not smoking in front of children or grandchildren.
- Explain that stopping smoking will enhance both quantity and quality of life expectancy, and give examples of things that giving up smoking would allow the smoker to do.
- Highlight the importance of attending behavioural support sessions and using pharmacotherapy; encourage smokers to use both.
- Discuss potential nicotine withdrawal symptoms and explain that although these are at their worst in the first few days, most will pass within about a month.
- Emphasise the need to eat healthily and take regular exercise as weight gain is often a concern during smoking cessation.
- Explain that treatment with nicotine replacement therapy (NRT) or bupropion helps prevent weight gain.
- Encourage patients to create goals and rewards for themselves and highlight financial benefits of smoking cessation.
- Devise coping mechanisms to use during periods of craving.
- Give written information to support your advice, so that the risks of smoking and health benefits of quitting can be reinforced at home by family members.
- Deliver behavioural advice yourself, or ask a smoking cessation specialist (such as those available through National Health Service (NHS) smoking cessation services) to do it for you.
- Arrange to review all smokers, either personally or through a smoking cessation specialist, soon after the quit attempt. Use this review to monitor progress, employ alternative strategies if necessary and provide further support and encouragement.

Box 5.1 **Brief advice from health professional should be given to all smokers**

- The best thing you can do for your health is to stop smoking, and I advise you to stop as soon as possible. The sooner you stop the better.
- How do you feel about your smoking?
- How do you feel about tackling your smoking now?

Providing brief advice leads to 2-3% of smokers becoming long-term abstainers.

Box 5.2 **Behavioural strategies for smoking cessation**

- Set a quit date and tell friends and colleagues that you are quitting.
- Prepare by avoiding smoking in places you spend a lot of time in.
- Get rid of all cigarettes.
- Do not 'cut down' or 'have the odd one' – go for total abstinence.
- Review past attempts; look at what has helped and what has not.
- Anticipate challenges and think of ways of dealing with them.
- Encourage partners to quit at the same time and offer them support.
- Use nicotine replacement therapy, bupropion or varenicline.
- Make use of follow-up support.

Nicotine replacement therapy

NRT is the most commonly used cessation therapy and increases the chances of quitting by about 40% (nicotine gum) to 100% (nasal spray). NRT exerts its effects by replacing the supply of nicotine to the individual but without the toxic components of cigarette smoke. Many smokers incorrectly believe that nicotine is toxic.

NRT is available in many different formulations. Although some forms of NRT (gum, inhalator delivery, nasal spray or lozenges) deliver nicotine more quickly than others (transdermal patches), all deliver a lower total dose, and deliver it to the brain more slowly than a cigarette. Individuals should be offered a choice of different formulations of NRT, but the use of combination therapy with a transdermal patch to provide continuous background nicotine and a more rapidly acting product (lozenge, gum, inhalator or nasal spray) to use in advance of regular cigarette times and other times of particular craving is helpful. In individuals with relative contraindications (such as acute cardiovascular disease or pregnancy), it may be prudent to use lower doses of relatively short-acting preparations. Relatively light smokers (<10 cigarettes per day), or those who wait longer than an hour before their first cigarette of the day, may also be better advised to use a short-acting product in advance of their regular cigarettes or at times of craving.

Treatment is generally recommended for 10–12 weeks but smokers may continue to use NRT for longer if they feel they need it. There is no evidence to suggest that gradual withdrawal of NRT is better than abrupt withdrawal, although the former method is usually favoured. NRT products are generally well tolerated and side effects relatively minor (Box 5.3): cautions to NRT use are all relative and should always be overriden if the likely alternative is that the smoker will relapse into smoking.

Box 5.3 **Prescribing points with NRT**

- Adverse effects
  - Nausea
  - Headache
  - Unpleasant taste
  - Hiccoughs and indigestion
  - Sore throat
  - Nose bleeds
  - Palpitations
  - Dizziness
  - Insomnia
  - Nasal irritation (spray)
- Cautions
  - Hyperthyroidism
  - Diabetes mellitus
  - Renal and hepatic impairment
  - Gastritis and peptic ulcer disease
  - Peripheral vascular disease
  - Skin disorders (patches)
  - Avoid nasal spray when driving or operating machinery (sneezing, watering eyes)
  - Severe cardiovascular disease (arrhythmias, post-myocardial infarction)
  - Recent stroke
  - Pregnancy
  - Breastfeeding

Bupropion

Bupropion has similar efficacy as NRT in improving quit rates. It is an antidepressant but its effect on smoking cessation is independent of this property. Bupropion also helps prevent weight gain. The most important adverse effect recognised with bupropion is an association with convulsions; the drug is therefore contraindicated in those with a past history of epilepsy and seizures. Bupropion should not generally be prescribed in individuals with other risk factors for seizures and some drugs – such as antidepressants, antimalarials, antipsychotics, quinolones and theophylline – can lower the seizure threshold.

Unlike NRT – which is usually started at the same time as quitting smoking – it is recommended that bupropion is commenced in advance of the quit date, by 1 or 2 weeks. Treatment is usually continued for 8 weeks. There is no clear evidence that combining bupropion with NRT confers any further advantage in quit rates. Indeed, doing so can lead to hypertension and insomnia.

Varenicline

Varenicline is a partial nicotine agonist, which also blocks nicotine receptors from stimulation by free nicotine. Varenicline is an effective smoking cessation oral drug, which increases the likelihood of quitting by a factor of about 2.3, and is thus slightly more effective than NRT or bupropion. There is no evidence that combining varenicline with other therapies is any more effective than varenicline alone. Like bupropion, varenicline should be started a week prior to the planned quit day, with increasing doses over the first few days. The most common side effect of varenicline is nausea. Some cases of depression and suicidal ideation in association with varenicline have been reported, suggesting that it is prudent to avoid the drug in patients at particular risk of these problems.

Implementing smoking cessation in routine care

One of the major barriers to smoking cessation practice is that many health professionals either do not have the skills and knowledge to intervene in smokers, and/or fail to intervene routinely in clinical practice. It is essential that determining smoking status, delivering brief advice and offering further help to smokers interested in quitting become routine practice throughout all medical disciplines, especially in patients with COPD (Box 5.4). Too many patients are still not offered the effective therapies that could help them to quit.

Box 5.4 **The five As of smoking cessation should form a routine component of all health service delivery**

- **Ask**   about tobacco use
- **Advise**   to quit
- **Assess**   willingness to make an attempt
- **Assist**   in quit attempt
- **Arrange**   follow-up

Further reading

Cahill K, Stead LF, Lancaster T. Nicotine receptor partial agonists for smoking cessation. *The Cochrane Database of Systematic Reviews* 2008; (3). Art. No.: CD006103. DOI: 10.1002/14651858.CD006103.pub3.

Hughes JR, Stead LF, Lancaster T. Antidepressants for smoking cessation. *The Cochrane Database of Systematic Reviews* 2007; (1). Art. No.: CD000031. DOI: 10.1002/14651858.CD000031.pub3.

National Institute for Health and Clinical Excellence. *Smoking Cessation Services in Primary Care, Pharmacies, Local Authorities and Workplaces, Particularly for Manual Working Groups, Pregnant Women and Hard to Reach Communities. NICE Public Health Guidance 10.* National Institute for Health and Clinical Excellence, London, 2008.

Stead LF, Perera R, Bullen C, Mant D, Lancaster T. Nicotine replacement therapy for smoking cessation. *The Cochrane Database of Systematic Reviews* 2008; (1). Art. No.: CD000146. DOI: 10.1002/14651858.CD000146.pub3

CHAPTER 6

Non-pharmacological Management

Graeme P. Currie and Graham Douglas

Aberdeen Royal Infirmary, Aberdeen, UK

OVERVIEW

- The multidisciplinary team plays an important role in the overall management of patients with chronic obstructive pulmonary disease (COPD)

- Pulmonary rehabilitation improves symptoms, exercise tolerance and quality of life, but has no impact on lung function or exacerbation frequency

- Influenza and pneumococcal vaccination should be offered to all patients

- Formal nutritional advice should be considered in overweight or underweight patients

- An attempt should be made to recognise and treat anxiety and depression, both of which often coexist with COPD

- Surgical approaches to COPD in carefully selected motivated individuals include bullectomy, lung volume reduction surgery and transplantation

---

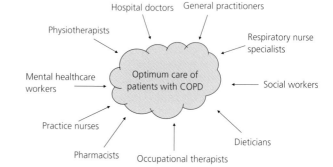

Figure 6.1 Multidisciplinary team input is required in most patients. COPD, chronic obstructive pulmonary disease.

Chronic obstructive pulmonary disease (COPD) is a slowly progressive and largely irreversible disorder. Pharmacological interventions alone are unable to ensure optimal outcomes (Box 6.1), and non-pharmacological strategies and multidisciplinary team input are increasingly important in overall management. Indeed, a broad spectrum of professionals from both primary and secondary care should be involved, with the aim of delivering optimum care that is individualised to the patient (Figure 6.1). Many of these healthcare professionals can greatly assist patients with the medical, physical, domestic and social limitations posed by severe breathlessness to function successfully in the community.

Box 6.1 **Treatment aims of COPD**

- Reduce symptoms and exacerbations.
- Improve lung function.
- Improve exercise tolerance.
- Improve health-related quality of life.
- Provide care satisfactory to the patients' needs.
- Provide a treatment regime, which minimises the risk and frequency of adverse effects.
- Reduce mortality.
- Prevent or slow down disease progression.

Pulmonary rehabilitation

Pulmonary rehabilitation can be defined as 'a multidisciplinary programme of care for patients with chronic respiratory impairment that is individually tailored and designed to optimise physical and social performance and autonomy'. Unfortunately, it is only currently available for a small proportion of patients who would benefit from it, although community-based programmes are becoming more common. Pulmonary rehabilitation is instrumental in breaking the self-perpetuating vicious circle that patients with COPD frequently encounter (Figure 6.2). Other factors such as immobility, hypoxia, malnutrition, increased oxidative stress and systemic inflammation may all contribute towards skeletal muscle atrophy and in turn reduce exercise capacity and heighten fatigue.

In addition to assessing and advising on dysfunctional breathing and helping airway clearance, physiotherapists play an important role in pulmonary rehabilitation programmes. Although the duration, setting and format of pulmonary rehabilitation varies, a typical outpatient session may run for 6–8 weeks with supervised exercise occurring 2–3 times a week. Depending on local availability, most functionally impaired patients with COPD – irrespective of age and smoking status – should be offered pulmonary rehabilitation. However, some will find participation difficult because of time

---

ABC of COPD, 2nd edition.
Edited by Graeme P. Currie. © 2011 Blackwell Publishing Ltd.

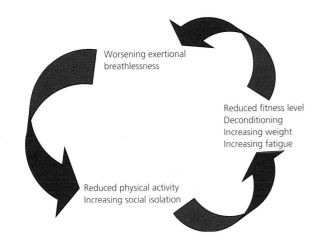

Figure 6.2 A determined attempt should be made to break the vicious circle of worsening breathlessness, reduced physical activity and deconditioning.

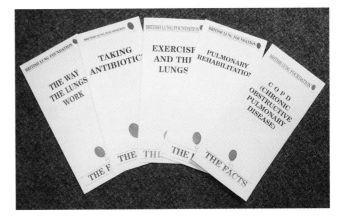

Figure 6.3 Educating patients about chronic obstructive pulmonary disease (COPD) plays an important role in management.

constraints, travel and hospital parking implications and motivational issues. The ideal programme should include exercise training, education and nutritional support.

Long-term outcomes of pulmonary rehabilitation

Improvements in exercise performance and reduced exercise-associated breathlessness can be maintained for up to 12 months. Pulmonary rehabilitation can also improve the quality of life, although this benefit tends to decline over time. However, there is no influence on disease progression (as judged by decline in forced expiratory volume in 1 second (FEV_1)), exacerbation frequency or long-term survival. Data regarding healthcare utilisation are conflicting, with no consistent reduction in hospital admission rates or length of hospital stay being observed. Community pulmonary rehabilitation immediately following an exacerbation of COPD can lead to improvements in exercise capacity and overall health status.

Exercise training

Exercise training should involve the muscles of walking, in addition to strength training of upper and lower limbs. Patients are encouraged to exercise at home and complete records so that progress can be monitored; a minimum of thrice weekly 30-minute periods of moderate exercise is a reasonable starting level. There are few absolute contraindications to exercise, although unstable angina, severe aortic stenosis, uncontrolled hypertension, recent myocardial infarction, severe peripheral vascular disease and major mobility problems are examples. Studies have shown that physiological changes provided by endurance training take place at the level of skeletal muscle, even during submaximal exercise. Regular exercise training can lead to improvements in

- exercise tolerance;
- symptoms;
- quality of life;
- peak oxygen uptake;
- endurance time during submaximal exercise;
- walking distance;
- peripheral and respiratory muscle strength.

Education

Patient education in pulmonary rehabilitation covers various forms of goal-directed and systematically applied communication, directed at improving understanding and motivation (Figure 6.3). The education programme should be provided in a structured way and potential topics include breathing control, relaxation, benefits of exercise, going on holiday, causes and treatments of COPD, review of available allowances and value of smoking cessation. Although education individualised to the patient is often helpful, group-based education may be more effective. Participants are encouraged to take responsibility for their own health and follow-up sessions may be necessary at home. Many other useful techniques can be taught during pulmonary rehabilitation sessions (Table 6.1, Figure 6.4) and these may help in reducing symptoms during periods of increased activity or an exacerbation.

Nutritional advice

Many patients with COPD are underweight and malnourished. Increased calorific requirement because of increased work of breathing, reduced nutritional intake due to limitations posed

Table 6.1 Different techniques which may reduce breathlessness and allow more efficient ventilation.

Technique	Instruction and effects
Pursed lip breathing	May reduce respiratory rate and aid recovery during periods of increased activity
Relaxed, slower, deeper breathing	May allow more effective ventilation during exertion and avoid rapid shallow breathing
Paced breathing	Timing inhalation and exhalation with every other breath may help reduce symptoms during activity
Positioning	Passive fixing of the shoulder girdle (e.g. elbows resting on a table or ledge) may reduce breathlessness. Patients should also be encouraged to adopt the forward lean sitting position
Energy-conservation technique	Home adaptations (such as a hand rail) or sitting to perform household chores
Exhalation on effort	Advise patients to exhale when they perform an activity (such as standing up, lifting the arms)

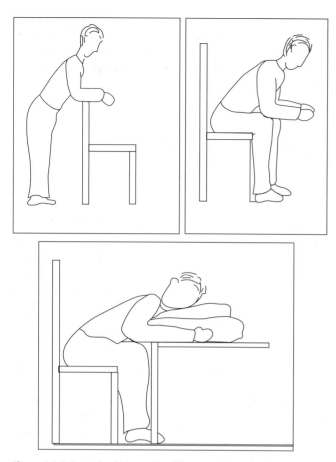

Figure 6.4 Patients should be taught different positions which use less energy and may help reduce work of breathing.

by severe breathlessness and chronic systemic inflammation are all factors in weight loss. In contrast, some patients become overweight partly because of reduced activity, social isolation and overeating. The prevalence of obesity in COPD is higher than in the general population. The reasons for these differences are unclear, although elevated levels of cytokines such as tumour necrosis factor-α and leptin have been implicated in weight loss. Moreover, being underweight and weight loss are independent risk factors for a poorer prognosis. The body mass index (BMI; Box 6.2) should be calculated in all patients with COPD, and is now a component in the calculation of the BODE (**B**MI, **O**bstruction, **D**yspnoea and **E**xercise) index (see Chapter 3).

Formal dietary advice can be helpful in individuals who are underweight (BMI <18.5) or obese (BMI >30). A Cochrane review of the effects of nutritional supplementation in COPD failed to demonstrate any significant impact upon lung function or exercise capacity, although the quality, numbers and size of studies included were suboptimal. However, in one recent study, dietary counselling and food fortification did result in weight gain in nutritionally 'at-risk' patients along with improvement in quality of life and levels of activity. Whether long-term gains from nutritional supplementation can be sustained is uncertain and further work is required to determine whether other therapies such as the use of creatine and hormones (which increase muscle mass) provide worthwhile benefits.

Box 6.2 **Calculation and categorisation of body mass index**

- BMI = weight (in kilograms) divided by the height^2 (in metres)
- For example, in a 70 kg patient who is 1.7 metres tall,
  ○ BMI = 70 / (1.7)^2
  ○ BMI = 24
- The BMI in Europeans can be categorised as follows:
  ○ Underweight: <18.5
  ○ Normal weight: 18.5–24.9
  ○ Overweight: 25–29.9
  ○ Obesity: 30–39.9
  ○ Morbid obesity: ≥40
  ○ In Asians, corresponding values are <18.5, 18.5–22.9, 23–24.9, 25–29.9 and ≥30 respectively.

BMI, body mass index.

Immunisation

Many exacerbations of COPD are caused by viruses and bacteria, with the implication that prevention of infection by way of vaccination might play an important role. Current guidelines indicate that unless contraindications exist, annual influenza and single pneumococcal immunisation should be offered to all patients with COPD. Over the past two decades, an increasing number of patients have been immunised against both influenza and pneumococcus (Figures 6.5 and 6.6).

Pneumococcal vaccination

Current pneumococcal vaccines contain purified capsular polysaccharide from each of 23 subtypes of *Streptococcus pneumoniae*. A single dose of 0.5 ml is given intramuscularly and mild soreness and induration at the site of injection is a common occurrence. Reimmunisation is not advised and is contraindicated within 3 years. Severe reactions to reimmunisation probably occur because

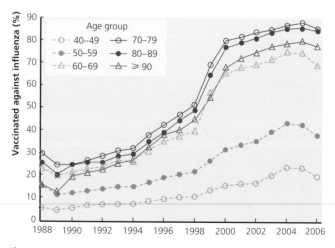

Figure 6.5 Trends in vaccination rates against influenza in patients aged >40 years with chronic obstructive pulmonary disease. Figure reproduced with permission from Schembri S, Morant S, Winter JH, MacDonald TM. Influenza but not pneumococcal vaccination protects against all-cause mortality in patients with COPD. *Thorax* 2009; **64**: 567–572.

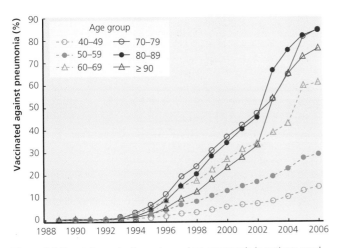

Figure 6.6 Trends in vaccination rates against pneumonia in patients aged >40 years with chronic obstructive pulmonary disease. Figure reproduced with permission from Schembri S, Morant S, Winter JH, MacDonald TM. Influenza but not pneumococcal vaccination protects against all-cause mortality in patients with COPD. *Thorax* 2009; **64**: 567–572.

of high levels of circulating antibodies. Recent data have suggested that pneumococcal vaccination reduces invasive pneumococcal disease including pneumonia, with no effect on all-cause mortality.

Influenza vaccination

Influenza vaccine is prepared each year using viruses (usually two type A and one type B subtypes) similar to those considered most likely to be circulating in the forthcoming winter (Figure 6.7). The viruses are grown in the allantoic cavity of chick embryos and the vaccine is therefore contraindicated in individuals with egg allergy. Patients are often concerned about adverse effects and doubts may exist about the protective efficacy of the vaccine. A Cochrane meta-analysis of 20 cohort studies evaluating the effects

of inactivated influenza vaccination in high-risk patients (including some with COPD) confirmed that inactivated vaccine did confer an overall reduction in exacerbation rates. In another meta-analysis of individuals receiving influenza vaccination, the pooled estimates of efficacy for patients over 65 years of age were

- 56% for preventing respiratory illness;
- 53% for preventing pneumonia;
- 50% for preventing hospital admission;
- 68% for preventing death.

Anxiety and depression

Anxiety and depression often coexist in patients with COPD and are under-recognised and undertreated. Moreover, concomitant depression may be associated with poorer quality of life, reduced survival, persistent smoking, higher hospital admission rate and more symptoms. The presence of anxiety or depression in patients with COPD has also been directly associated with the severity of airflow obstruction. All this suggests that interventions that reduce anxiety and depression should be considered where necessary. These conditions are likely to be multifactorial in origin, with social isolation, persistent symptoms and inability to easily participate in activities of daily living all playing a role.

Clinical features suggestive of an anxiety or depressive disorder should be positively sought in all patients with COPD; one simple way of assessing this is by the hospital anxiety and depression scale (Box 6.3). The presence of tiredness, low energy, weight loss and poor sleep are fairly non-specific and often occur in both COPD and depression. If anxiety or depression is likely to be present, cognitive behavioural approaches along with conventional drug treatments are therapeutic options, although robust evidence suggesting that they have a positive impact on COPD are lacking. In depression, tricyclic antidepressants or selective serotonin reuptake inhibitors should be considered, whereas in anxiety, selective serotonin reuptake inhibitors and benzodiazepines are options. If benzodiazepines are prescribed, clinicians should be vigilant for respiratory depression and oversedation. An aggressive attempt to optimise lung function and treat significant hypoxaemia should also be undertaken in these patients.

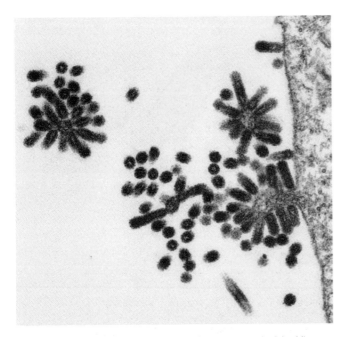

Figure 6.7 Electron micrograph showing influenza viruses (red) budding from a host cell. Reproduced with permission from sciencephoto.com.

Box 6.3 **Hospital anxiety and depression scale**

Anxiety

- I feel tense or wound up
  Most of the time – 3, a lot of the time – 2, from time to time – 1, not at all – 0
- I get a sort of frightened feeling as if something awful is going to happen
  Definitely and badly – 3, yes, but not too badly – 2, a little – 1, not at all – 0
- Worrying thoughts go through my mind
  Very definitely – 3, yes, but not too badly – 2, a little – 1, not at all – 0
- I can sit at ease and feel relaxed
  Definitely – 0, usually – 1, not often – 2, not at all – 3

- I get a sort of frightened feeling like butterflies in the stomach
  Not at all – 0, occasionally – 1, quite often – 2, very often – 3
- I feel restless as if I have to be on the move
  Very much indeed – 3, quite a lot – 2, not very much – 1, not at all – 0
- I get sudden feelings of panic
  Very often indeed – 3, quite often – 2, not very often – 1, not at all – 0

Depression

- I look forward with enjoyment to things
  As much as I ever did – 0, rather less than I used to – 1, definitely less than I used to – 2, hardly at all – 3
- I have lost interest in my appearance
  Definitely – 3, I take not so much care as I should – 2, I may not take quite as much care – 1, I take as much care as ever – 0
- I still enjoy the things I used to enjoy
  Definitely as much – 0, not quite so much – 1, only a little – 2, hardly at all – 3
- I can laugh and see the funny side of things
  As much as I always could – 0, not quite so much – 1, definitely not so much – 2, not at all – 3
- I feel cheerful
  Not at all – 3, not often – 2, sometimes – 1, most of the time – 0
- I feel as if I am slowed down
  Nearly all the time – 3, very often – 2, sometimes – 1, not at all – 0
- I can enjoy a good book, the radio or a TV programme
  Often – 0, sometimes – 1, not often – 2, seldom – 3

Scoring is based on a 4-point scale (0–3). A score of 0–7 is normal, 8–10 borderline and 11–21 suggests moderate-to-severe anxiety or depression

Surgery

Some patients with COPD will need to undergo emergency and elective surgical procedures and prior risk assessment is usually necessary. Having a diagnosis of COPD is associated with an increased post-operative complication rate of three to fivefold, although the further the procedure is from the diaphragm, the lower this risk becomes. Optimising lung function along with smoking cessation 1–2 months before surgery should be strongly encouraged, as doing so may reduce this risk even further. Following surgery, a determined attempt at early post-operative mobilisation should be made along with deep breathing techniques, intermittent positive pressure breathing, measures to reduce the chance of developing thromboembolism and effective analgesia.

A small number of patients with COPD should be considered for a surgical procedure to the lungs in an attempt to improve lung function and quality of life. However, given their increased operative and post-operative risk and the frequency of co-morbidities (such as ischaemic heart disease), surgical approaches should only be considered in motivated former smokers who have significant symptoms despite maximal treatment. The three most common

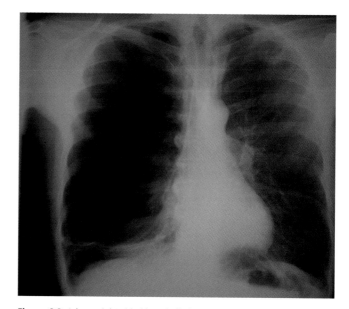

Figure 6.8 A large right-sided lung bulla in a patient with chronic obstructive pulmonary disease (COPD).

procedures undertaken are bullectomy, lung volume reduction surgery (LVRS) and transplantation.

Bullectomy

In some patients with COPD, bullae can occupy large volumes of the chest cavity, causing compression of surrounding functional lung parenchyma (Figure 6.8). Bullectomy thereby allows decompression of the less affected lung. In symptomatic patients with a single large bulla, especially those with moderate-to-severe airflow obstruction, previous pneumothorax or haemoptysis, bullectomy should be considered. Other factors that should prompt consideration of bullectomy include normal blood gases, FEV_1 >40% predicted and normal or near-normal gas transfer. This procedure is less likely to be of benefit in those with advanced emphysematous change in the remaining lung, pulmonary hypertension and hypercapnia. Bullectomy may improve lung function, symptoms and quality of life.

It is important to note that when admitted to hospital, differentiating a pneumothorax from a large bulla can frequently be difficult and computed tomographic (CT) imaging may be necessary. Inadvertent chest drain insertion into a bulla can lead to complications such as bronchopleural fistula.

Lung volume reduction surgery

Lung volume reduction surgery (LVRS) aims to remove areas of inefficient emphysematous lung parenchyma, thereby promoting better gas exchange in the less affected part. LVRS can improve quality of life, exercise capacity and lung function in carefully selected individuals, and in subgroup analysis of some studies, prolong survival. Moreover, it is safer than transplantation and avoids the problem of lack of donor lungs. Which patients benefit most from this procedure is not fully established, although LVRS should be considered in patients fulfilling the following criteria:

- Predominantly upper lobe disease
- Significant functional impairment despite maximal pharmacological treatment and pulmonary rehabilitation
- $pO_2 > 6\,kPa$ and $pCO_2 < 8\,kPa$
- $FEV_1 < 45\%$ predicted
- Physiological features of hyperinflation

Recently, there has been interest in bronchoscopic lung volume reduction in patients with COPD. This involves obstructing emphysematous areas of lung with an endobronchial valve, thereby avoiding risks of major surgery. The role of this new procedure requires further evaluation.

Lung transplantation

Some motivated former smokers with COPD should be considered for lung transplantation, although, as in most transplant procedures, this is greatly limited by organ availability. Patients with co-morbidities and advanced age generally have poorer survival rates. The upper age limit for bilateral lung transplant is 60 years and for single lung transplant it is 65 years. Local guidelines should be consulted, although suggested criteria for referral include patients with a combination of

- advanced airflow obstruction ($FEV_1 < 25\%$ predicted);
- significant functional impairment despite maximal pharmacological treatment and pulmonary rehabilitation;
- cor pulmonale and pulmonary hypertension;

- hypercapnia;
- suspected prognosis of <2 years.

Further reading

Bott J, Blumenthal S, Buxton M *et al*. Joint BTS/ACPRC guideline: guidelines for the physiotherapy management of the adult, medical, spontaneously breathing patient. *Thorax* 2009; **64**(suppl 1): i1–i52.

British Thoracic Society Guidelines. Pulmonary rehabilitation. *Thorax* 2001; **56**: 827–834.

Ferreira IM, Brooks D, Lacasse Y, Goldstein RS. Nutritional support for individuals with COPD: a meta-analysis. *Chest* 2000; **117**: 672–678.

Fishman A, Martinez F, Naunheim K *et al*. A randomized trial comparing lung-volume-reduction surgery with medical therapy for severe emphysema. *New England Journal of Medicine* 2003; **348**: 2059–2073.

Gross PA, Hermogenes AW, Sacks HS, Lau J, Levandowski, RA. The efficacy of influenza vaccine in elderly persons. A meta-analysis and review of the literature. *Annals of Internal Medicine* 1995; **123**: 518–527.

Hopkinson NS, Toma TP, Hansell DM *et al*. Effect of bronchoscopic lung volume reduction on dynamic hyperinflation and exercise in emphysema. *American Journal of Respiratory and Critical Care Medicine* 2005; **171**: 453–460.

Man WD, Polkey MI, Donaldson N, Gray BJ, Moxham J. Community pulmonary rehabilitation after hospitalisation for acute exacerbations of chronic obstructive pulmonary disease: randomised controlled study. *British Medical Journal* 2004; **329**: 1209.

Poole PJ, Chacko E, Wood-Baker RWB, Cates CJ. Influenza vaccine for patients with chronic obstructive pulmonary disease. *The Cochrane Database of Systematic Reviews* 2006; CD002733.

Weekes CE, Emery PW, Elia M. Dietary counselling and food fortification in stable COPD: a randomised trial. *Thorax* 2009; **64**: 326–331.

Wilson I. Depression in the patient with COPD. *International Journal of COPD* 2006; **1**: 61–64.

CHAPTER 7

Pharmacological Management (I) – Inhaled Treatment

Graeme P. Currie[1] *and Brian J. Lipworth*[2]

[1]Aberdeen Royal Infirmary, Aberdeen, UK
[2]Asthma and Allergy Research Group, Ninewells Hospital and Medical School, Dundee, UK

OVERVIEW

- All patients with chronic obstructive pulmonary disease (COPD) should use a short-acting bronchodilator (short-acting β_2-agonist or short-acting anticholinergic) for as required relief of symptoms

- A long-acting bronchodilator (long-acting anticholinergic or long-acting β_2-agonist) should be started in those with persistent symptoms and exacerbations if the FEV_1 is $\geq$50% of predicted

- Inhaled corticosteroids play no role as monotherapy in COPD

- A long acting β_2-agonist plus inhaled corticosteroid or long acting anticholinergic should be considered in patients with persistent symptoms and exacerbations who have an $FEV_1 <$ 50% of predicted

- A long-acting anticholinergic, long-acting β_2-agonist and inhaled corticosteroid should be used in patients with advanced disease who have persistent symptoms and exacerbations

---

Chronic obstructive pulmonary disease (COPD) is a heterogeneous condition and all patients should be regarded as individuals. This is apparent not only in terms of presentation, natural history, symptoms, disability and frequency of exacerbations but also in response to treatment. The stepwise titration of pharmacological therapy in COPD is usually based around

- extent of airflow obstruction;
- severity of symptoms (usually breathlessness);
- functional limitation;
- presence and frequency of exacerbations.

Physiological effects of inhaled bronchodilators

It is increasingly apparent that inhaled bronchodilators confer important clinical benefits over and above changes in forced expiratory volume in 1 second (FEV_1). Relying upon measures of lung function alone to monitor the effects of bronchodilators may be a rather simplistic approach, and has the potential to miss important physiological and clinical benefits. Air trapping, which

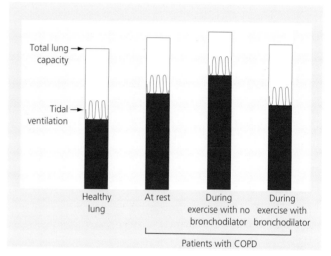

Figure 7.1 Patients with chronic obstructive pulmonary disease (COPD) have pulmonary hyperinflation with an increased functional residual capacity (purple) and a decreased inspiratory capacity (white). This increases the volume at which tidal breathing (oscillating line) occurs and places the muscles of respiration at mechanical disadvantage. Hyperinflation worsens with exercise and therefore reduces exercise tolerance (dynamic hyperinflation). Inhaled bronchodilators improve dynamic hyperinflation, in addition to hyperinflation at rest, thereby reducing the work of breathing and increasing exercise tolerance.

is manifested clinically as hyperinflation, is frequently found in patients with advanced COPD; this places the respiratory muscles at a mechanical disadvantage. During exercise, air trapping increases even further, which in turn perpetuates the mechanical disadvantage experienced at rest (Figure 7.1). Inhaled bronchodilators reduce measures of air trapping at rest and on exercise (static and dynamic hyperinflation), which may well occur without significant changes in FEV_1. Moreover, as COPD is largely an irreversible condition, relying solely on outcome measures such as lung function may result in potentially important beneficial effects being missed upon parameters such as static lung volumes, quality of life and exacerbation frequency.

Short-acting bronchodilators

Short-acting β_2-agonists such as salbutamol and terbutaline act directly upon bronchial smooth muscle to dilate the airway

---

Table 7.1 Pharmacological properties of the main inhaled bronchodilators used in COPD.

Class	Drug	Onset (minutes)	Peak effect (minutes)	Duration (hours)
Short-acting β_2-agonist	Salbutamol	5	60–90	4–6
	Terbutaline	5	60–90	4–6
Long-acting β_2-agonist	Formoterol	5	60–90	12
	Salmeterol	45–60	120–240	12
Short-acting anticholinergic	Ipratropium	5–15	60–120	4–6
Long-acting anticholinergic	Tiotropium	15	60–240	36

(Table 7.1). This class of drug reduces breathlessness, improve lung function and are effective when used on an 'as required basis'.

Short-acting anticholinergics such as ipratropium offset high-resting bronchomotor vagally induced tone and also dilate the airways. These drugs have been shown in some studies to reduce breathlessness, improve lung function, improve health-related quality of life and reduce the need for rescue mediation.

All patients with COPD should therefore be prescribed a short-acting inhaled bronchodilator (β_2-agonist or anticholinergic) for as required relief of symptoms. Patients using the long-acting anticholinergic tiotropium should *not* be prescribed a short-acting anticholinergic, but rather a short-acting β_2-agonist for as required use.

Long-acting bronchodilators

In COPD, the two classes of inhaled long-acting bronchodilator available are long-acting anticholinergics (tiotropium) and long-acting β_2-agonists (formoterol and salmeterol). Numerous studies have evaluated their effects in COPD, and guidelines indicate that a long-acting bronchodilator as monotherapy should be given to symptomatic patients with an $FEV_1 \geq 50\%$ of predicted. If symptoms persist thereafter, both classes of long-acting bronchodilator may be used concurrently through separate inhaler devices. Long-acting anticholinergics and long-acting β_2-agonists are usually well tolerated, although adverse effects do occur in some patients (Box 7.1).

Box 7.1 **Adverse effects of long-acting bronchodilators**

- Long-acting β_2-agonists
  - Tachycardia
  - Fine tremor
  - Headache
  - Muscle cramps
  - Prolongation of the QT interval
  - Hypokalaemia
  - Feeling of nervousness
- Long-acting anticholinergics
  - Dry mouth
  - Nausea
  - Constipation
  - Headache
  - Tachycardia
  - Acute angle glaucoma
  - Bladder outflow obstruction

Long-acting anticholinergics

Airflow obstruction in COPD is multifactorial in origin and is in part due to potentially reversible high cholinergic tone. Moreover, mechanisms mediated by the vagus nerve are implicated in enhanced submucosal gland secretion in patients with COPD. This knowledge has led to the development of a long-acting once-daily administered anticholinergic drug (tiotropium).

Three main subtypes (M_1, M_2 and M_3) of muscarinic receptors exist. The activation of both M_1 and M_3 receptors results in bronchoconstriction whereas the M_2 receptor is protective against such an effect. In contrast to ipratropium, tiotropium dissociates rapidly from the M_2 receptor (therefore minimising the loss of any putative benefit) and dissociates only slowly from the M_3 receptor. This in turn causes a reduction in resting bronchomotor tone, smooth muscle relaxation and airways dilation for a greater length of time. In the United Kingdom, it is the only licensed long-acting anticholinergic and can be delivered via a breath-activated dry powder inhaler (Handihaler) or soft mist inhaler (Respimat).

Numerous studies of patients with COPD have shown tiotropium to be more effective than both placebo and ipratropium. This is in terms of lung function, symptoms, quality of life and exacerbations. In a meta-analysis of nine studies, tiotropium was associated with a reduction in exacerbations and hospital admissions compared to placebo and ipratropium. In the same study, tiotropium was significantly better at improving lung function than long-acting β_2-agonists. In the study by Tashkin *et al.* (2008), the effects of add-on tiotropium to all other medication were evaluated over a 4-year period in nearly 6000 patients with an FEV_1 of <70% of predicted. Compared to placebo, tiotropium was associated with improvements in lung function, health-related quality of life, mortality and exacerbations, although it failed to reduce the overall rate of decline in FEV_1; a subgroup analysis, however, indicated that in patients with less advanced disease (mean FEV_1 59% predicted), tiotropium did slow the rate in lung function decline (Figure 7.2). The mechanism by which tiotropium reduces exacerbations is unclear, but it may be due to sustained bronchodilation preventing a fall in lung function during infective episodes.

Long-acting β_2-agonists

Long-acting β_2-agonists act directly upon β_2-adrenoceptors causing smooth muscle to relax and airways to dilate. The two most widely used drugs – formoterol and salmeterol – are given on a twice daily basis. In contrast to short-acting β_2-agonists, both salmeterol and formoterol are relatively lipophilic (fat soluble) and have prolonged receptor occupancy. Factors such as these may in part explain their prolonged duration of action. *In vitro* data have shown that formoterol more potently relaxes smooth muscle compared to salmeterol.

A Cochrane systematic review of 23 trials evaluating the effects of long-acting β_2-agonists demonstrated that salmeterol produced modest increases in lung function and a consistent reduction in exacerbations, although variable effects for other outcomes such as health-related quality of life or symptoms were observed.

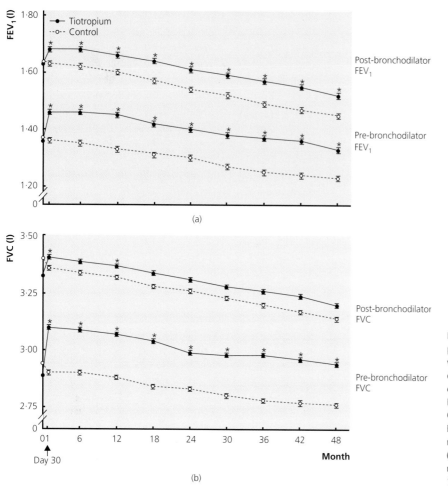

(a)

(b)

Day 30

Month

Figure 7.2 Effects of add-on tiotropium on mean pre- and post-bronchodilator forced expiratory volume in 1 second (FEV_1) (a) and forced vital capacity (FVC) (b) in patients with less advanced chronic obstructive pulmonary disease (COPD). Reproduced with permission from Decramer M, Celli B, Kesten S, Lystig T, Mehra S, Tashkin DP. Effect of tiotropium on outcomes in patients with moderate chronic obstructive pulmonary disease (UPLIFT): a prespecified subgroup analysis of a randomised controlled trial. *Lancet* 2009; **374**: 1171–1178.

Combinations of long-acting anticholinergic *plus* long-acting β₂-agonist

Several studies have evaluated the effects of a long-acting anticholinergic plus long-acting β_2-agonist (formoterol and salmeterol) in combination. In one study, tiotropium plus formoterol resulted in greater improvements in lung function than either agent alone. In another study, tiotropium when added to salmeterol, failed to improve lung function, exacerbation frequency or need for hospital admission.

Inhaled corticosteroids

Commonly prescribed inhaled corticosteroids include beclomethasone dipropionate, budesonide and fluticasone propionate. It is important to note that many patients with COPD – even those with minimal symptoms and mild airflow obstruction – have been treated in the past with inhaled corticosteroids as monotherapy. This is despite the relative insensitivity of corticosteroids upon the neutrophlic inflammation found in COPD and paucity of evidence showing significant short- or long-term benefits. Historically, this is due to clinicians incorrectly extending the beneficial role of anti-inflammatory treatment in asthma to that of

COPD, along with a lack of alternative pharmacological strategies previously available. Indeed, the exact role of inhaled corticosteroids in the management of COPD has been a contentious issue over the past few decades and several large multicentre studies and meta-analysis have attempted to address this uncertainty.

It is fairly well established that inhaled corticosteroids as monotherapy do not have any appreciable impact upon reducing the rate of decline in FEV_1 (Figure 7.3) or mortality. In one large study by Burge *et al.* (2000), 1000 μg/day of fluticasone did confer a 25% reduction in exacerbations, with most benefit being observed in patients with mean $FEV_1 < 50\%$ predicted. In other studies, there have been inconsistent effects upon secondary end points, with either no or only small improvements in symptoms and quality of life. In a Cochrane meta-analysis in 2007 evaluating >13,000 individuals, long-term inhaled corticosteroids failed to reduce the decline in FEV_1 and no beneficial effects upon mortality were observed. Treatment was, however, associated with reductions in the mean rate of exacerbations per year and rate of decline in quality of life. The dose of inhaled corticosteroid required to achieve maximal beneficial effect with minimal adverse effect (optimum therapeutic ratio) is uncertain. Current evidence

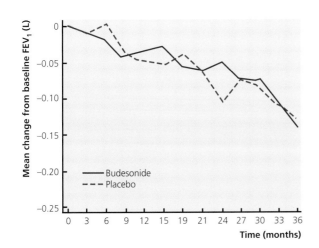

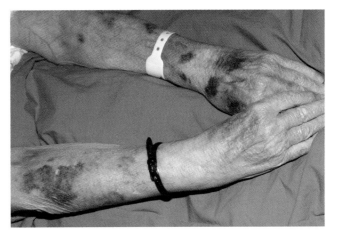

Figure 7.3 Inhaled corticosteroids have not been shown to influence the rate in decline in lung function in chronic obstructive pulmonary disease (COPD). In this study of patients with mild COPD, no difference in mean change in baseline forced expiratory volume in 1 second (FEV_1) between placebo and budesonide was observed over 36 months. Reproduced with permission from Vestbo *et al. Lancet* 1999; **353**: 1819–1823.

Figure 7.5 Extensive skin bruising in a patient using inhaled corticosteroids.

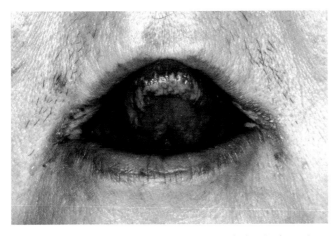

Figure 7.4 Oropharyngeal candidiasis in a patient with chronic obstructive pulmonary disease (COPD) using high-dose inhaled corticosteroids.

suggests that inhaled corticosteroids should be prescribed in patients with an FEV_1 < 50% predicted and who experience frequent (>2 per year) exacerbations.

Adverse effects of inhaled corticosteroids

Inhaled corticosteroids cause both local and systemic adverse effects. Common local adverse sequelae include oropharyngeal candidiasis (Figure 7.4) and dysphonia. Previous studies have shown that skin bruising (Figure 7.5) occurs more commonly in patients using inhaled corticosteroids and variable effects have been observed in reduction of bone mineral density and suppression of the hypothalamic–pituitary–adrenal axis. Moreover, the TORCH trial by Calverley *et al.* (2007) demonstrated an increased risk of pneumonia in patients receiving inhaled corticosteroids alone and when used in conjunction with a long-acting β_2-agonist.

Combined inhaled corticosteroid plus long-acting β_2-agonist inhalers

Most studies evaluating long-acting β_2-agonists and inhaled corticosteroids have shown superiority with the combination product over the single agent alone. For example, in the largest study evaluating this combination of drugs (TORCH), fluticasone plus salmeterol in combination was better than either drug as monotherapy in terms of survival, FEV_1, exacerbation frequency and quality of life over a 3-year period. In studies evaluating the combination of budesonide with formoterol, the proportion of reductions in exacerbations (25%) were similar to the TORCH study with the combination product versus placebo. In most studies evaluating long-acting β_2-agonists and inhaled corticosteroids in combination, the mean FEV_1 was <50% predicted. In the study by Wedzicha *et al.* (2008), the combination of fluticasone plus salmeterol was compared to tiotropium. Exacerbation rates were similar in both groups, although pneumonia was more common and mortality was lower with the combination treatment. Combined inhaled corticosteroid plus long-acting β_2-agonist inhalers are licensed for use in the United Kingdom when individuals have an FEV_1 < 60% predicted and >2 exacerbations annually.

Triple therapy

In advanced symptomatic COPD, many patients are prescribed a combination of a long-acting anticholinergic, a long-acting β_2-agonist and an inhaled corticosteroid. This approach has not been fully evaluated and only few studies have involved patients using such triple therapy. In two studies by Tashkin *et al.* (2008) and Welte *et al.* (2009), the addition of tiotropium to fluticasone plus salmeterol resulted in a reduction in exacerbations in one study, but not the other. However, in another study, the addition of tiotropium to formoterol plus budesonide compared to tiotropium alone did result in greater improvements in lung function, health status, symptoms and reduction in severe exacerbations (Figure 7.6).

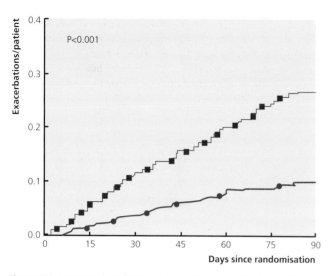

Figure 7.6 Mean number of severe exacerbations per patient versus time with tiotropium plus placebo (purple squares) versus tiotropium plus budesonide/formoterol (blue circles). Reproduced with permission from Welte T, Miravitlles M, Hernandez P *et al.* Efficacy and tolerability of budesonide/formoterol added to tiotropium in COPD patients. *American Journal of Respiratory and Critical Care in Medicine* 2009; **180**: 741–750. (The authors would like to thank AstraZeneca for funding the copyright fee in order to reproduce this figure.)

It seems reasonable to continue to prescribe all three classes of drug in patients with more advanced airflow obstruction who have repeated exacerbations and persistent symptoms. However, it may well be that 'a ceiling effect' in terms of exacerbations exists and the effects of the individual components are less than additive.

Summary of inhaled treatment

Since airflow obstruction is the universal feature of clinically significant COPD, bronchodilators play an integral role in all stages of disease. In all symptomatic patients with COPD, a short-acting inhaled bronchodilator should be used on an 'as required basis'.

In patients with persistent symptoms and exacerbations, updated NICE guidelines have suggested that regular inhaled drugs (alone or in combination) should be given depending on the FEV_1 percentage predicted (Figure 7.7).

If the FEV_1 is ≥50% of predicted, options include a once-daily long-acting anticholinergic or twice-daily long-acting β_2-agonist. If symptoms and exacerbations persist, options include both a long-acting anticholinergic plus long-acting β_2-agonist or long-acting β_2-agonist plus inhaled corticosteroid. Evidence for the latter approach is weak, and combined inhalers (containing a long-acting β_2-agonist plus corticosteroid) must be prescribed within the drug licence.

If the FEV_1 is <50% of predicted, options include a once-daily anticholinergic as monotherapy or long-acting β_2-agonist plus inhaled corticosteroid (as a combination inhaler). If symptoms and exacerbations persist, all three classes of inhaled drug should be considered. In all stages of disease, patients should be made aware of the potential risk of developing side effects (including non-fatal pneumonia) when using inhaled corticosteroids.

Algorithm for use of inhaled therapies.

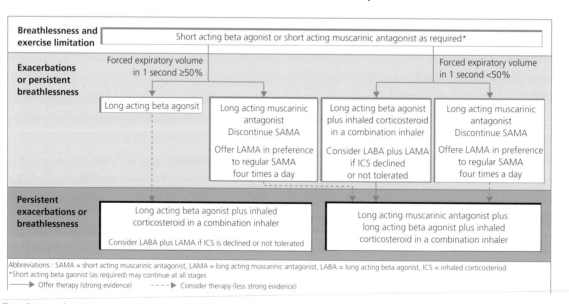

Figure 7.7 Flow diagram showing suggested algorithm for inhaled drug treatment in patients with chronic obstructive pulmonary disease (COPD). FEV_1, forced expiratory volume in 1 second. Figure reproduced with permission from O'Reilly J, Jones MM, Parnham J, Lovibond K, Rudolf M. Management of stable chronic obstructive pulmonary disease in primary and secondary care: summary of updated NICE guidance. *BMJ* 2010; **340**:c3134.

Further reading

Aaron SD, Vandemheen KL, Fergusson D *et al.* Tiotropium in combination with placebo, salmeterol, or fluticasone–salmeterol for treatment of chronic obstructive pulmonary disease: a randomized trial. *Annals of Internal Medicine* 2007; **146**: 545–555.

Appleton S, Poole P, Smith B, Veale A, Lasserson TJ, Chan MM. Long-acting β$_2$-agonists for chronic obstructive pulmonary disease patients with poorly reversible airflow limitation. *The Cochrane Database of Systematic Reviews* 2006 July 19; **3**: CD001104.

Barr RG, Bourbeau J, Camargo CA, Ram FS. Tiotropium for stable chronic obstructive pulmonary disease: a meta-analysis. *Thorax* 2006; **61**: 854–862.

Calverley PM, Boonsawat W, Cseke Z, Zhong N, Peterson S, Olsson H. Maintenance therapy with budesonide and formoterol in chronic obstructive pulmonary disease. *European Respiratory Journal* 2003; **22**: 912–919.

Celli B, Decramer M, Kesten S, Liu D, Mehra S, Tashkin DP. Mortality in the 4 year trial of tiotropium (UPLIFT) in patients with COPD. *American Journal of Respiratory and Critical Care Medicine* 2009; **180**: 948–955.

Decramer M, Celli B, Kesten S, Lystig T, Mehra S, Tashkin DP. Effect of tiotropium on outcomes in patients with moderate chronic obstructive pulmonary disease (UPLIFT): a prespecified subgroup analysis of a randomised controlled trial. *Lancet* 2009; **374**: 1171–1178.

Sin DD, Tashkin D, Zhang X *et al.* Budesonide and the risk of pneumonia: a meta-analysis of individual patient data. *Lancet* 2009; **374**: 712–719.

Szafranski W, Cukier A, Ramirez A *et al.* Efficacy and safety of budesonide/formoterol in the management of chronic obstructive pulmonary disease. *European Respiratory Journal* 2003; **21**: 74–81.

van Noord JA, Aumann JL, Janssens E *et al.* Comparison of tiotropium once daily, formoterol twice daily and both combined once daily in patients with COPD. *European Respiratory Journal* 2005; **26**: 214–222.

Yang IA, Fong KM, Sim EH, Black PN, Lasserson TJ. Inhaled corticosteroids for stable chronic obstructive pulmonary disease. *The Cochrane Database of Systematic Reviews* 2007 April 19; (2): CD002991.

References

Burge PS, Calverley PMA, Jones PW, Spencer S, Anderson JA, Maslem TK. Randomised, double blind, placebo controlled study of fluticasone propionate in patients with moderate to severe chronic obstructive pulmonary disease: the ISOLDE trial. *BMJ* 2000; **320**: 1297–1303.

Calverley PMA, Anderson JA, Celli B *et al.* and the TORCH investigators. Salmeterol and fluticasone propionate and survival in chronic obstructive pulmonary disease. *New England Journal of Medicine* 2007; **356**: 775–789.

Tashkin DP, Celli B, Senn S *et al.* A 4-year trial of tiotropium in chronic obstructive pulmonary disease. *New England Journal of Medicine* 2008; **359**: 1543–1554.

Wedzicha JW, Calverley PMA, Seemungal TA, Hagan G, Ansari Z, Stockley RA for the INSPIRE investigators. The prevention of chronic obstructive pulmonary disease exacerbations by salmeterol/fluticasone propionate or tiotropium bromide. *American Journal of Respiratory and Critical Care Medicine* 2008; **177**: 19–26.

Welte T, Miravitlles M, Hernandez P *et al.* Efficacy and tolerability of budesonide/formoterol added to tiotropium in COPD patients. *American Journal of Respiratory and Critical Care Medicine* 2009; **180**: 741–750.

CHAPTER 8

Pharmacological Management (II) – Oral Treatment

Graeme P. Currie[1] *and Brian J. Lipworth*[2]

[1] Aberdeen Royal Infirmary, Aberdeen, UK
[2] Asthma and Allergy Research Group, Ninewells Hospital and Medical School, Dundee, UK

OVERVIEW

- No clinically useful or effective oral bronchodilator without significant adverse effects exists for patients with chronic obstructive pulmonary disease (COPD)

- Theophylline – a weak bronchodilator and anti-inflammatory agent – has a limited role in the management of stable COPD; low doses may confer benefit by activation of histone deacetylase and potentiate the anti-inflammatory activity of corticosteroids

- Roflumilast – a new, once-daily selective phosphodiesterase-4 inhibitor – is an anti-inflammatory agent which reduces exacerbations of COPD and produces small improvements in lung function additive to long-acting inhaled bronchodilators; adverse effects include gastrointestinal disturbance, headache and weight loss

- No evidence exists indicating that long-term oral corticosteroids are of benefit in COPD and should be avoided if possible

- The role of mucolytics is not clear, although they may reduce exacerbation frequency in some patients not using inhaled corticosteroids

- Long-term antibiotics and antitussives are not indicated in COPD

Inhaled treatment forms the cornerstone of pharmacological management in chronic obstructive pulmonary disease (COPD). However, some individuals – especially the elderly, those with cognitive impairment and upper limb musculoskeletal problems – experience technical difficulties with, and are unable to consistently and successfully use, inhaler devices. Unfortunately, there are fairly significant unmet needs in terms of effective orally active, long-acting bronchodilator therapy in COPD, and no major advances in this respect have taken place over the past few decades. However, a number of oral drugs can be considered in different circumstances in a selected number of individuals.

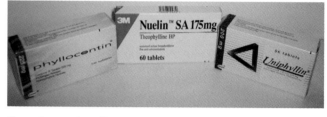

Figure 8.1 A variety of long-acting theophylline preparations are available and are usually given to patients in a twice-daily dosing regime.

Theophylline

Theophylline is one of the oldest oral therapeutic agents available for the treatment of COPD (Figure 8.1). It shares a chemical structure similar to that of caffeine, which is also a bronchodilator in large amounts. Theophylline is a non-selective phosphodiesterase (PDE) inhibitor which results in an increase in the level of intracellular cyclic adenosine monophosphate (cAMP) in a variety of cell types and organs (including the lungs). Increases in cAMP levels are implicated in inhibitory effects upon inflammatory and immunomodulatory cells. One of the end results is that PDE inhibition causes relaxation of smooth muscle and dilatation of the airway. However, a number of other potentially beneficial mechanisms of action of theophylline in COPD have been suggested. These include

- reduction of diaphragmatic muscle fatigue;
- increased mucociliary clearance;
- respiratory centre stimulation;
- inhibition of neutrophilic inflammation;
- suppression of inflammatory genes by activation of histone deacetylases;
- inhibition of cytokines and other inflammatory cell mediators;
- potentiation of anti-inflammatory effects of inhaled corticosteroids at low doses (via increased histone deacetylase activity);
- potentiation of bronchodilator effects of β_2-agonists.

Clinical use of theophylline

Over the years, theophylline has been used less extensively because of limited efficacy, narrow therapeutic index, commonly encountered adverse effects and interactions with many other drugs. However, a

ABC of COPD, 2nd edition.
Edited by Graeme P. Currie. © 2011 Blackwell Publishing Ltd.

long-acting theophylline should still be considered in patients with more advanced COPD, especially when symptoms persist despite the use of other treatments or when patients are unable to use inhaler devices. Various studies have demonstrated that theophylline does generally confer small benefits in lung function (as reflected by the forced expiratory volume in 1 second (FEV_1) and forced vital capacity (FVC) when combined with different classes of inhaled bronchodilators (anticholinergics and β_2-agonists) (Figure 8.2). In a meta-analysis of 20 randomised controlled trials involving patients of variable COPD severity, theophylline also conferred small overall improvements in FEV_1 (100 ml) and arterial blood gas tensions compared to placebo, although the incidence of nausea was significantly higher with active drug. The slow onset of action of theophylline – combined with the necessary dose titration to achieve suitable plasma levels – means that benefit may not be observed until after several weeks. As with most drugs in COPD, clinicians should discontinue it if a therapeutic trial is unsuccessful. It has recently been suggested that lower doses of theophylline than that previously used may still confer benefit, perhaps because of enhanced activity of histone deacetylase (and increased corticosteroid sensitivity in smokers) and suppression of inflammation.

Adverse effects

One of the main limitations preventing more extensive prescribing of theophylline is its capacity to cause dose-dependent adverse effects (Box 8.1), in addition to numerous patient characteristics and drugs that alter its half-life (Box 8.2). The plasma concentration of theophylline should be checked when initially titrating the dose upwards, or when adding in a new drug that may alter its metabolism. Target levels are between 10 and 20 mg/l (55–110 μM), which reflect the bronchodilator window, whereas lower levels are associated with anti-inflammatory and histone deacetylase activity. At theophylline concentrations greater than this, the frequency of adverse effects tends to increase to an unacceptable extent. During an exacerbation, the dose of theophylline should be reduced by 50% if a macrolide (e.g. clarithromycin) or fluoroquinolone (e.g. ciprofloxacin) is prescribed.

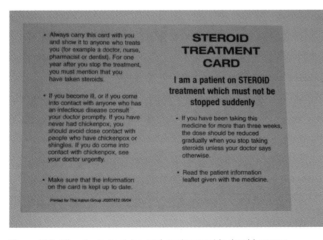

Figure 8.2 All patients receiving oral corticosteroids should carry a treatment card at all times.

Box 8.1 Adverse effects of theophylline

- Tachycardia
- Cardiac arrhythmias
- Nausea and vomiting
- Abdominal pain
- Diarrhoea
- Headache
- Irritability and insomnia
- Seizures
- Hypokalaemia

Box 8.2 Drugs and patient characteristics which alter the plasma theophylline concentration

- Causes of increased plasma theophylline levels (i.e. reduced plasma clearance)
  - Heart failure
  - Liver cirrhosis
  - Advanced age
  - Ciprofloxacin
  - Erythromycin
  - Clarithromycin
  - Verapamil
- Causes of reduced plasma theophylline levels (i.e. increased plasma clearance)
  - Cigarette smokers
  - Chronic alcoholism
  - Rifampicin
  - Phenytoin
  - Carbamazepine
  - Lithium

A group of more selective PDE4 inhibitors have been developed in an attempt to confer benefit with fewer adverse effects than theophylline. One of the most advanced PDE4s is roflumilast. This drug is given once daily, but is associated with adverse effects such as nausea, diarrhoea, headache and weight loss. It acts mainly as an anti-inflammatory agent to reduce exacerbations and has a small effect on FEV_1 when used with a long-acting bronchodilator. There are no head-to-head studies comparing theophylline and roflumilast. The role of roflumilast in COPD remains to be established, especially as it is not known if it confers additive anti-inflammatory effects to combination therapy with inhaled corticosteroid and long-acting β_2-agonist.

Oral corticosteroids

Although there is increasing evidence that COPD is associated with an abnormal systemic inflammatory response, oral corticosteroids have a limited role in the management of stable disease. Despite their long-term use in some patients, there is little or no evidence supporting this practice, while discontinuation of long-term systemic corticosteroids in steroid-dependent patients has not been shown to cause a significant increase in COPD exacerbations. Moreover, oral corticosteroids have unwanted effects on skeletal muscle and diaphragmatic function, which may well compound existing respiratory muscle weakness. As a general rule, long-term corticosteroids should be avoided. Guidelines do acknowledge that there are some severely symptomatic patients with advanced airflow obstruction in whom it is difficult to discontinue corticosteroids following an exacerbation, although this may well in part be due to mood-enhancing effects. In situations where withdrawal is impossible, the lowest possible dose (e.g. 5 mg/day prednisolone) should be considered.

Prevention of corticosteroid-associated adverse effects

Before starting oral corticosteroids, patients should know the dose of drug to be taken, its anticipated duration and potential adverse effects (Figure 8.3). Individuals receiving long-term oral corticosteroids should be aware that they should not be stopped suddenly and that a slow reduction in dose is usually necessary. Immediate withdrawal after prolonged administration may lead to acute adrenal insufficiency and even death. As a consequence, all patients receiving oral corticosteroids should have a treatment card (Figure 8.2) alerting others on the problems associated with abrupt discontinuation. Courses of oral corticosteroids which last less than 3 weeks (e.g. given to treat an exacerbation of COPD) do not generally require to be tapered before stopping.

The risk of corticosteroid-induced osteoporosis is related to cumulative dose (Figures 8.4 and 8.5). This implies that in addition to individuals receiving maintenance prednisolone, those requiring frequent courses may experience long-term complications. Patients using at least 7.5 mg/day of prednisolone (or equivalent) for 3 months are at heightened risk of adverse effects along with those over the age of 65 years.

Bisphosphonates reduce the rate of bone turnover and are therefore useful in the prevention and treatment of corticosteroid-related osteoporosis. Dual energy X-ray absorptiometry (DEXA) scans can facilitate early identification of patients at risk of corticosteroid-associated adverse effects and

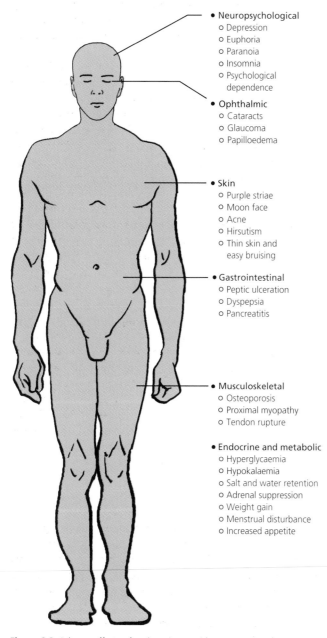

- **Neuropsychological**
  - o Depression
  - o Euphoria
  - o Paranoia
  - o Insomnia
  - o Psychological dependence
- **Ophthalmic**
  - o Cataracts
  - o Glaucoma
  - o Papilloedema
- **Skin**
  - o Purple striae
  - o Moon face
  - o Acne
  - o Hirsutism
  - o Thin skin and easy bruising
- **Gastrointestinal**
  - o Peptic ulceration
  - o Dyspepsia
  - o Pancreatitis
- **Musculoskeletal**
  - o Osteoporosis
  - o Proximal myopathy
  - o Tendon rupture
- **Endocrine and metabolic**
  - o Hyperglycaemia
  - o Hypokalaemia
  - o Salt and water retention
  - o Adrenal suppression
  - o Weight gain
  - o Menstrual disturbance
  - o Increased appetite

Figure 8.3 Adverse effects of oral corticosteroids.

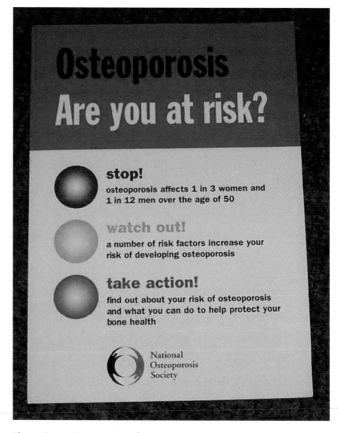

Figure 8.4 Patients receiving frequent courses of, or maintained on, long-term oral corticosteroids should be aware of the risks of osteoporosis. Such patients should ensure an adequate intake of dietary calcium and be encouraged to exercise. Post-menopausal women should consider using hormone replacement therapy.

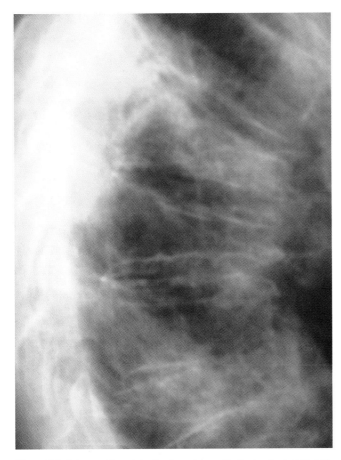

Figure 8.5 Osteoporotic vertebral collapse in a patient using long-term oral corticosteroids; this elderly patient was not using a bisphosphonate.

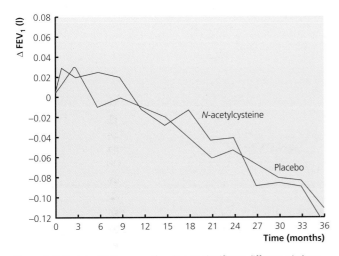

Figure 8.6 Kaplein–Meijer curve showing no significant difference in lung function in patients receiving N-acetyl cysteine and placebo. Figure reproduced with permission from Decramer et al. Effects of N-acetylcysteine on outcomes in chronic obstructive pulmonary disease (Bronchitis Randomized on NAC Cost-Utility Study, BRONCUS): a randomised placebo-controlled trial. *Lancet* 2005; **365**: 1552–1560. FEV$_1$, forced expiratory volume in 1 second.

are frequently requested in patients attending specialist clinics. They also highlight which patients should ensure adequate calcium intake and vitamin D3, and where necessary commence a weekly bisphosphonate (e.g. risedronate or alendronate). Patients who have previously sustained a low-velocity fracture (Figure 8.6) should be started on treatment for osteoporosis if oral corticosteroids are used on a long-term basis. Irrespective of bone density, a regular bisphosphonate should be started on initiation of long-term corticosteroids in individuals aged over 65 years.

Mucolytics

Excessive lower respiratory tract secretions and sputum overproduction are commonly found in patients with COPD. Mucolytics are thought to reduce the viscosity of sputum in the airways and help patients expectorate, while they may also confer some benefit by way of antioxidant effects. Indeed, in a meta-analysis of 23 studies, regular mucolytic treatment reduced the frequency of exacerbations by 29% without significant improvement in lung function. However, a major limitation was that many of the patients involved had chronic bronchitis rather than COPD.

In one study by Zheng *et al.* (2008) in Chinese patients with COPD who had a mean FEV$_1$ < 50% predicted (of whom only around 20% were using bronchodilators and inhaled corticosteroids), 1500 mg/day of carbocysteine significantly reduced exacerbations over a 1-year period compared to placebo. In another study, Bronchitis Randomized On NAC Cost-Utility Study (BRONCUS), where most patients (mean FEV$_1$ 57% predicted) were using inhaled corticosteroids and long-acting bronchodilators, 600 mg/day of N-acetyl cysteine failed to prevent deterioration in lung function, prevent exacerbations or improve health-related quality of life (Figures 8.6 and 8.7) over 3 years. In a subgroup analysis, those who were not receiving inhaled corticosteroids did, however, experience fewer exacerbations.

Two mucolytic agents that are currently licensed for use in the United Kingdom are carbocysteine and mecysteine hydrochloride; both are generally well tolerated, although they should be used with caution in those with peptic ulceration as they may disrupt the gastric mucosal barrier. These agents may be considered in patients with cough productive of sputum, who experience frequent exacerbations, although further data are required to fully delineate their place in COPD management and they should not be routinely used. Erdosteine is another mucolytic which may be considered for up to 10 days of an acute exacerbation of COPD.

Other drugs

Regular long-term antibiotics are not indicated in the prophylaxis of exacerbations and doing so may only encourage the emergence of strains of bacteria that are resistant to conventional broad-spectrum antibiotics. While there are few data supporting their widespread use in stable COPD, regular low-dose erythromycin has been shown to reduce the number of exacerbations (perhaps due to anti-inflammatory activity) compared to placebo over a 12-month period.

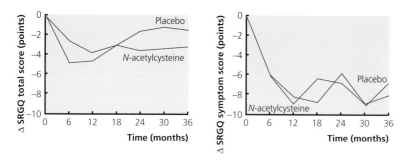

Figure 8.7 Kaplein–Meijer curves showing no significant difference in health status, measured with St George's respiratory questionnaire, in patients receiving *N*-acetyl cysteine and placebo. Figure reproduced with permission from Decramer *et al.* Effects of *N*-acetylcysteine on outcomes in chronic obstructive pulmonary disease (Bronchitis Randomized on NAC Cost-Utility Study, BRONCUS): a randomised placebo-controlled trial. *Lancet* 2005; **365**: 1552–1560.

Cough is frequently a troublesome symptom in many patients, although it may, in fact, be advantageous, especially in patients who produce copious amounts of sputum. Antitussives are not known to provide any benefit in COPD, other than perhaps short-term symptomatic control of cough; their regular use should be discouraged.

In patients with cor pulmonale, there is little or no evidence that drugs such as angiotensin-converting enzyme inhibitors, digoxin or calcium channel blockers are of benefit. If measures such as leg elevation and compression stockings – and, where appropriate, long-term oxygen therapy – fail to control symptomatic peripheral oedema, low-dose diuretics can be tried. In such circumstances, renal function should be carefully monitored.

Further reading

Barnes PJ. Theophylline: new perspectives on an old drug. *American Journal of Respiratory and Critical Care Medicine* 2003; **167**: 813–818.

Calverley PM, Rabe KF, Goehring UM, Kristiansen S, Fabbri LM, Martinez FJ. Roflumilast in symptomatic chronic obstructive pulmonary disease: two randomised clinical trials. *Lancet* 2009; **374**: 685–694.

Cosio BG, Iglesias A, Rios A *et al.* Low-dose theophylline enhances the anti-inflammatory effects of steroids during exacerbations of COPD. *Thorax* 2009; **64**: 424–429.

Decramer M, Molken MR, Dekhuijzen PN *et al.* Effects of N-acetylcysteine on outcomes in chronic obstructive pulmonary disease (Bronchitis Randomized on NAC Cost-Utility Study, BRONCUS): a randomised placebo-controlled trial. *Lancet* 2005; **365**: 1552–1560.

Fabbri LM, Calverley PM, Izquierdo-Alonso JL *et al.* Roflumilast in moderate-to-severe chronic obstructive pulmonary disease treated with long-acting bronchodilators: two randomised clinical trials. *Lancet* 2009; **374**: 695–703.

Lipworth BJ. Phosphodiesterase-4 inhibitors for asthma and chronic obstructive pulmonary disease. *Lancet* 2005; **365**: 167–175.

Poole PJ, Black PN. Oral mucolytic drugs for exacerbations of chronic obstructive pulmonary disease: systematic review. *British Medical Journal* 2001; **322**: 1271–1274.

Ram FSF, Jones PW, Castro AA *et al.* Oral theophylline for chronic obstructive pulmonary disease. *The Cochrane Database of Systematic Reviews* 2002; (3). Art. No.: CD003902.

Rice KL, Rubins JB, Lebahn F *et al.* Withdrawal of chronic systemic corticosteroids in patients with COPD: a randomized trial. *American Journal of Respiratory and Critical Care Medicine* 2000; **162**: 174–178.

Seemungal TA, Wilkinson TM, Hurst JR, Perera WR, Sapsford RJ, Wedzicha JA. Long-term erythromycin therapy is associated with decreased chronic obstructive pulmonary disease exacerbations. *American Journal of Respiratory and Critical Care Medicine* 2008; **178**: 1139–1147.

Walters JAE, Walters EH, Wood-Baker R. Oral corticosteroids for stable chronic obstructive pulmonary disease. *The Cochrane Database of Systematic Reviews* 2005; (2). CD005374.

References

Zheng JP, Kang J, Huang SG *et al.* Effect of carbocisteine on acute exacerbation of chronic obstructive pulmonary disease (PEACE Study): a randomised placebo-controlled study. *Lancet* 2008; **371**: 2013–2018.

CHAPTER 9

Inhalers

Graeme P. Currie and Graham Douglas

Aberdeen Royal Infirmary, Aberdeen, UK

> **OVERVIEW**
>
> - Inhaler technique is often neglected in the overall care of patients with chronic obstructive pulmonary disease (COPD)
> - Patients should be given specific instruction on use of the particular inhaler and be able to use it with confidence
> - Inhaler technique should be assessed at every available opportunity as technique declines over time
> - A pressurised metered dose inhaler (pMDI) should ideally be used with a compatible spacer
> - Dry powder inhalers (DPIs) reduce the need for coordination and are easier to use than pMDIs
> - If a patient is unable to use a particular device, an alternative should be considered
> - Bronchodilators delivered by nebuliser may be considered in those with persistent severe symptoms and advanced airflow obstruction (who demonstrate subjective and/or objective benefit), and those unable to use inhalers correctly

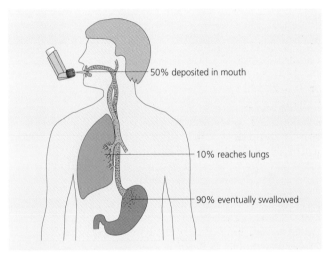

50% deposited in mouth

10% reaches lungs

90% eventually swallowed

Figure 9.1 Only a small amount of the drug leaving a metered dose inhaler reaches the lungs.

Drugs have been administered by inhalation for thousands of years. For example, between 2000 and 1500 BC in Egypt and India, herbal preparations were burned and the vapours inhaled. Over subsequent years, a variety of medicinal and non-medicinal substances have been inhaled as treatments for breathlessness, and eventually a primitive nebuliser was developed in the mid-1800s. In 1929, the potential benefits of inhaled adrenaline were reported for patients with obstructive lung disorders and pressurised metered dose inhalers (pMDIs) were introduced in the 1950s.

Most drugs used in chronic obstructive pulmonary disease (COPD) are orally inhaled using hand-held devices. This makes intuitive sense as this route of delivery means that drugs are delivered topically to the airways. Unfortunately, only a small proportion of drug reaches the lungs, as a considerable amount is deposited in the mouth, throat and vocal cords and subsequently swallowed (Figure 9.1). This problem is accentuated with pMDIs, as difficulties are often encountered with coordinating actuation and inhalation. Further issues leading to suboptimal delivery are found in older patients; in those with impaired grip and movement of the hands or arms (e.g. in arthritis); the visually impaired and those who have difficulty in memorising, learning and retaining new information. Moreover, concordance (in both 'real-life' and clinical studies) with most inhaled devices is frequently far from ideal.

An increasingly bewildering array of inhaler devices is now available and problems often arise for both the clinician and patient as to which type should be prescribed. Moreover, many advantages and disadvantages of different inhaler types exist (Table 9.1). Evidence suggests that as many as 50% of patients fail to correctly use their inhaler sufficiently well to derive benefit from the prescribed drug. No perfect inhaler exists, but desirable attributes are shown in Box 9.1.

> Box 9.1 **Attributes of the ideal inhaler**
>
> - Ease of use during an acute episode of breathlessness
> - Ease of use as maintenance treatment
> - Easy to learn how to use
> - Quick delivery of drug
> - Portable, lightweight, hygienic and discreet
> - Moisture resistant

ABC of COPD, 2nd edition.
Edited by Graeme P. Currie. © 2011 Blackwell Publishing Ltd.

- Same type of inhaler for different drugs
- Ability to tell that a dose has been taken
- A dose counter to reflect how many inhalations remain
- No unpleasant local effects/taste
- Effective delivery of drug to the endobronchial tree
- Inexpensive
- Harmless to the environment
- Easily refillable
- Little or no maintenance or cleaning required

Choosing the correct inhaler

Studies have shown that different inhaler types can be equally effective in different groups of patients. When prescribing an inhaler, the overriding principles should be a combination of

- ability of the patient to use the device correctly and consistently;
- adequate instruction given by someone skilled in doing so;
- ability to switch to an alternative and more suitable device if necessary;
- patient preference;
- ease of use.

It is important that assessment and correction of inhaler technique is carried out at every available opportunity, as over time patients often become less able to use their inhaler correctly.

Different types of inhalers

Metered dose inhaler

The most common inhaler device is a pMDI (Figure 9.2). Patients often have difficulty in using pMDIs, particularly coordinating actuation of the device with adequate inspiratory effort. Other common errors in the use of pMDIs include failure to exhale before actuation, too short a breath-hold following inspiration, and too rapid an inspiratory flow. Moreover, radiolabelled studies have shown that only around 10% of the emitted drug – even with good technique – reaches the lungs. To correctly use a pMDI, patients should be asked to carry out the following steps:

- Remove the mouthpiece cover (if there is one) and shake the inhaler.
- Breathe out fully.
- Put your lips firmly around the mouthpiece.
- Press *only once* with the inhaler in your mouth and at the same time breathe inwards fully and deeply.
- Hold your breath for up to 10 seconds or as long as you find it comfortable.
- Breathe out normally.
- Repeat these steps if a second puff is required.
- Wipe the mouthpiece clean and replace its protective cover.

Some patients develop oropharyngeal candidiasis and complain of an alteration in the voice quality (dysphonia) when using a

Table 9.1 Advantages and disadvantages of different types of inhaler devices.

Type of inhaler	Advantages	Disadvantages
Metered dose inhaler	<ul><li>Portable</li><li>Inexpensive</li><li>Can be used quickly</li><li>Short treatment time</li><li>Contain high numbers of doses</li></ul>	<ul><li>Actuation and inhalation coordination required</li><li>Cold freon effect</li><li>High potential for poor technique</li><li>Usually no dose counter</li></ul>
Metered dose inhaler with spacer	<ul><li>More effective drug delivery</li><li>Reduced oropharyngeal drug deposition</li><li>No cold freon effect</li><li>Useful in emergency situations</li></ul>	<ul><li>Bulky</li><li>Maintenance/priming required to overcome electrostatic charges</li><li>Less portable</li><li>Education required for correct use</li><li>Additional cost of spacer</li><li>Usually no dose counter</li></ul>
Dry powder inhalers (Turbohaler, Accuhaler and Handihaler)	<ul><li>No actuation/inhalation coordination necessary</li><li>Portable</li><li>May have a dose counter</li><li>Spacer unnecessary</li><li>Short treatment time</li></ul>	<ul><li>Adequate inspiratory flow required</li><li>More expensive than pMDIs</li><li>No propellant</li><li>Should not be stored in damp environments</li></ul>
Breath-activated metered dose inhalers (Easibreathe and Autohaler)	<ul><li>No actuation/inhalation coordination necessary</li><li>Portable</li><li>Short treatment time</li></ul>	<ul><li>Cold freon effect</li><li>Adequate inspiratory flow required</li></ul>
Slow mist inhalers (Respimat)	<ul><li>Portable</li><li>Effective with smaller drug doses</li></ul>	<ul><li>No propellant</li><li>Actuation and inhalation coordination required (less than a pMDI)</li></ul>
Nebuliser	<ul><li>Tidal breathing adequate</li><li>Easy to use</li><li>Patient preference</li></ul>	<ul><li>Less portable, noisy and indiscreet</li><li>Expensive and maintenance required</li><li>Unpredictable lung deposition</li><li>Variable performance</li><li>Drug wastage</li><li>Long drug delivery time</li><li>Need for a power source</li></ul>

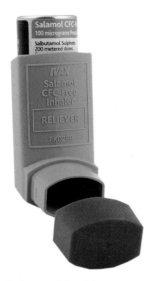

Figure 9.2 A pressurised metered dose inhaler.

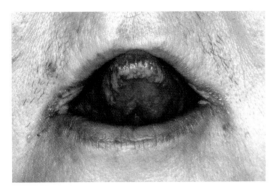

Figure 9.3 Oropharyngeal candidiasis in a patient receiving high dose inhaled corticosteroids.

pMDI to deliver inhaled corticosteroids (Figure 9.3). The risk of developing these problems can be minimised by gargling with water and mouth rinsing after pMDI use or using a spacer device to facilitate less upper airway deposition.

Metered dose inhaler plus spacer

A spacer device attached to a pMDI helps avoid problems in coordinating the timing of actuation and inhalation (Figure 9.4). It also overcomes the 'cold freon' effect whereby the cold blast of propellant reaching the oropharynx results in cessation of inhalation or inhalation through the nose (usually less of a problem

in inhalers using hydrofluouroalkane (HFA) compared to older chlorofluorocarbon (CFC) propellants). If used correctly, a pMDI with spacer is at least as effective for delivery of inhaled drugs as any other device. Different manufacturers make different sizes of spacers and inhalers, although the following principles of use can be applied to most types:

- Ensure the inhaler fits snugly into the end of the spacer device.
- Breathe out fully.
- Put your lips around the mouthpiece.
- Press the inhaler once.
- Breath inwards fully and deeply.
- Hold your breath for up to 10 seconds or as long as you find it comfortable (alternatively take five normal breaths in and out).
- Repeat these steps if a second puff is required.
- Wipe the mouthpiece clean.

Aerosol drug particles delivered into a spacer may become lost to the chamber walls by electrostatic attraction between drug particles and the chamber wall. This problem may be reduced by priming the chamber 10–20 times or washing it. Spacers should generally be cleaned at least once a month with soapy water and left to drip dry. They should be replaced every 6–12 months, depending on the manufacturer's recommendations.

Dry powder inhalers

Dry powder inhalers (DPIs) used in COPD – examples include Accuhalers, Turbohalers and the Handihaler – are all breath activated. This means that the inspiratory flow rate generated by the patient de-aggregates the powder into smaller particles which are then dispersed within the lungs. The need for coordination is less than when using a pMDI without a spacer and the DPIs are also less bulky and more portable. Different DPIs require different inspiratory flow rates (and higher flow rates than pMDIs) meaning that a more forceful inhalation is required to deposit the drug within the lungs (Table 9.2). This in turn may influence the type of DPI prescribed to patients, especially in those with more advanced airflow obstruction, hyperinflated lungs at rest and poor inspiratory reserve. Problems encountered with DPIs include failure to exhale to residual volume before use, exhaling into the mouthpiece after inhaling, inadequate or no breath-hold, failure to hold the device upright and failure to inhale with sufficient force.

Accuhalers

Accuhalers (Figure 9.5) deliver short-acting β_2-agonists (SABAs), long-acting β_2-agonists (LABAs), inhaled corticosteroids (ICS) and

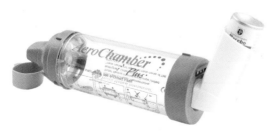

Figure 9.4 A metered dose inhaler with spacer.

Table 9.2 Minimum inspiratory flow rates required to use different types of inhalers.

Inhaler type	Minimum inspiratory flow rate (l/min)
Accuhaler	30
Turbohaler	30
Handihaler	20
Easibreathe inhaler	20–30
Autohaler	20–30

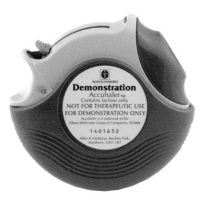

Figure 9.5 An Accuhaler.

LABAs and ICS in combination to the lungs. To use an Accuhaler correctly, patients should follow the following steps:

- Open the device by pressing down on the thumb rest.
- Click the lever down as far as possible.
- Breathe out fully.
- Put your lips around the mouthpiece and ensure a good seal.
- Breathe inwards fully and deeply.
- Hold your breath for up to 10 seconds or as long as you find comfortable.
- Wipe the mouthpiece clean and close the device.

Turbohalers

Turbohalers (Figure 9.6) deliver SABAs, LABAs, ICS and ICS in combination with LABAs to the lungs. To use a Turbohaler correctly, patients should be advised to take the following steps:

- Remove the outer cover.
- Hold the inhaler upright.
- Turn the base fully to the right and then back again until a click is heard.
- Breathe out fully.
- Put your lips around the mouthpiece and breathe inwards fully and deeply.
- Hold your breath for up to 10 seconds or as long as you find comfortable.
- Repeat these steps if a second puff is required.
- Wipe the mouthpiece clean and replace the outer cover.

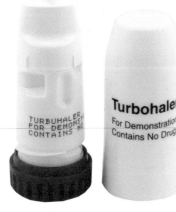

Figure 9.6 A Turbohaler.

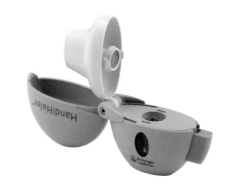

Figure 9.7 A Handihaler.

Handihaler

The Handihaler (Figure 9.7) delivers the long-acting anticholinergic drug tiotropium to the lungs. To use a Handihaler correctly, patients should be advised to take the following steps:

- Open the outer lid and inner white mouthpiece.
- Place a capsule into the inner basket.
- Press the button at the side of the inhaler once (this pierces the capsule).
- Breathe out fully.
- Put your lips around the mouthpiece and ensure a good seal.
- Breathe inwards fully and deeply.
- Hold your breath for up to 10 seconds or as long as you find it comfortable.
- Repeating these steps is often useful to ensure that most of the drug from within the capsule is used.
- Open the outer lid and mouthpiece and throw away the used capsule.
- Wipe the mouthpiece clean and replace the cap.

Breath-activated pMDIs

These types of inhalers were developed in an attempt to overcome some of the problems associated with pMDIs. When a patient inhales through the trigger device, a mechanism automatically 'fires' the breath-activated MDI with the subsequent release of drug. This means that inhalation and actuation coincide with one another.

Easibreathe inhalers

Easibreathe inhalers (Figure 9.8) deliver SABAs and ICS to the lungs. To use an Easibreathe inhaler correctly, patients should be advised to take the following steps:

- Shake the inhaler.
- Open the cap covering the mouthpiece.
- Breathe out fully.
- Put your lips around the mouthpiece and ensure a good seal (take care not to block the air holes).
- Breathe inwards fully and deeply.
- Hold your breath for up to 10 seconds or as long as you find comfortable.
- Repeat these steps if a second puff is required.
- Wipe the mouth piece clean and put the cap back over the mouthpiece.

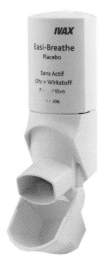

Figure 9.8 An Easibreathe inhaler.

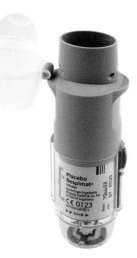

Figure 9.10 A Respimat inhaler.

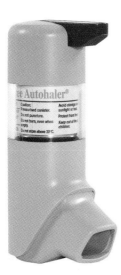

Figure 9.9 An Autohaler.

Autohalers

Autohalers (Figure 9.9) deliver SABAs and ICS to the lungs. To use an Autohaler correctly, patients should be advised to take the following steps:

- Shake the inhaler.
- Open the cap covering the mouthpiece.
- Breathe out fully.
- Put your lips around the mouthpiece and ensure a good seal (take care not to block the air holes).
- Breathe inwards fully and deeply.
- Hold your breath for up to 10 seconds or as long as you find comfortable.
- Repeat these steps if a second puff is required.
- Wipe the mouthpiece clean and replace the cap.

Soft mist inhalers

The Respimat (Figure 9.10) is the only soft mist inhaler currently available for use in COPD. It is a propellant-free inhaler and has been developed as an alternative device to the Handihaler to deliver tiotropium. It generates a mist with low spray momentum with small droplet size; 5 µg of tiotropium delivered via the Respimat is comparable to 18 µg delivered via the Handihaler. To use a Respimat inhaler correctly, patients should be advised to take the following steps:

- Hold the inhaler upright.
- Turn the base until it clicks.
- Open the transparent cap.
- Breathe out fully.
- Close lips around the end of the mouthpiece and direct the inhaler towards the back of the throat.
- Inhale slowly and deeply, and press the dose release button.

Nebulisers

Nebulisers are usually driven by compressed air but can be driven by oxygen if there is no history of hypercapnic respiratory failure. They create a mist of drug particles which is inhaled via a face mask or mouthpiece. Despite lack of objective benefit compared to the use of a pMDI with spacer, many patients express confidence in nebulisers, believe them to be more effective than other methods of drug delivery and are often the preferred (and requested) option.

Determining which patients should be prescribed a nebuliser to deliver bronchodilators in COPD is controversial. Indeed, with the introduction and increasing use of DPIs, the correct use of hand-held devices is within the grasp of many more patients. This in turn implies that fewer patients should be considered eligible for domiciliary nebulisers. However, it is reasonable to issue a nebuliser to patients with persistent and troublesome symptoms despite maximal treatment, although evidence of benefit should ideally be demonstrated. What actually qualifies as 'benefit' is far from clear, but may include a combination of reduction in breathlessness, improvement in exercise capacity, greater ability to perform daily living activities and improvement in lung function. Another indication is complete inability to correctly use or coordinate hand-held devices. Individuals using a nebuliser should receive adequate training and a facility for appropriate servicing and support should be available. Portable hand-held nebulisers of varying performance – in terms of drug delivery – are now also available.

Further reading

Broeders MEAC, Sanchis J, Levy ML, Crompton GK, Dekhuijzen PNR on behalf of the ADMIT Working Group. The ADMIT series – issues in inhalation therapy. 2) Improving technique and clinical effectiveness. *Primary Care Respiratory Journal* 2009; **18**: 76–82.

Jarvis S, Ind PW, Shiner RJ. Inhaled therapy in elderly COPD patients; time for re-evaluation? *Age and Ageing* 2007; **36**: 213–218.

Newman SP. Inhaler treatment options in COPD. *European Respiratory Review* 2005; **14**: 102–108.

Restrepo RD, Alvarez MT, Wittnebel LD *et al*. Medication adherence issues in patients treated for COPD. *International Journal of Chronic Obstructive Pulmonary Disease* 2008; **3**: 371–384.

CHAPTER 10

Oxygen

Graham Douglas and Graeme P. Currie

Aberdeen Royal Infirmary, Aberdeen, UK

OVERVIEW

- Normal oxygen saturation is between 95% and 98% in healthy adults breathing air at sea level

- Pulse oximeters are portable, non-invasive devices which assess oxygen saturation

- Giving high concentrations of oxygen to hypercapnic patients with COPD can lead to hypoventilation, a rise in $PaCO_2$ and development of acidosis

- The target SpO_2 should be 88–92% during an exacerbation of chronic obstructive pulmonary disease (COPD); the inspired oxygen concentration should be reduced if SpO_2 rises to >92%

- In hospital, patients with COPD who have normal pH and $PaCO_2$, the target SpO_2 is 94–98% (as loss of hypoxic drive is less likely)

- Long-term oxygen therapy (LTOT) is beneficial in patients with PaO_2 on air <7.3 kPa on two separate occasions or those with PaO_2 < 8 kPa with secondary polycythaemia, pulmonary hypertension, peripheral oedema or nocturnal hypoxaemia

- Ambulatory oxygen is increasingly available for patients who fulfil criteria for LTOT; it can be delivered by a small lightweight oxygen cylinder, liquid oxygen system or portable oxygen concentrator

- Conserving devices allow delivery of oxygen during inspiration but not in expiration; this leads to increased usage time and reduced cost of oxygen delivery

- There is little or no evidence that short burst oxygen confers benefit in patients with COPD

- In patients considering air travel, oxygen is not required if SpO_2 >95% and is required if SpO_2 <92%; those with SpO_2 92–95% should ideally have a hypoxic challenge test (breathing 15% oxygen)

In patients with chronic obstructive pulmonary disease (COPD), oxygen is used in a variety of settings. For example, it can be used at home, during transport to and from hospital and in hospital during an exacerbation. Administering oxygen is not without its dangers and it should be prescribed – in terms of flow rate and mode of

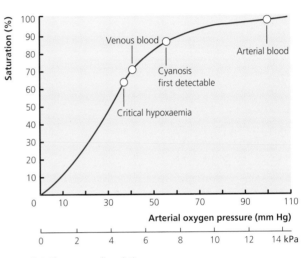

Figure 10.1 The oxygen dissociation curve.

delivery – like any other drug. All medical staff, nursing staff, and ambulance crews should be aware of the dangers of injudicious use of oxygen. At all times, it should therefore be considered whether it is actually necessary, and if so, what concentration and delivery device is most appropriate.

Oxygen physiology

Most circulating oxygen is bound to haemoglobin. As there is a fixed amount of haemoglobin, the amount of oxygen carried is usually expressed as the 'oxygen saturation' of haemoglobin. From an arterial sample, this is called SaO_2 and from a pulse oximeter, SpO_2. Alternatively, the oxygen tension or 'partial pressure of oxygen' (PaO_2) can be measured from an arterial sample of blood. The oxygen dissociation curve shows the relationship between oxygen saturation and arterial oxygen pressure (Figure 10.1). In healthy adults at sea level with normal PaO_2, SpO_2 is maintained between 95% and 98%.

Pulse oximetry

An oximeter is a spectrophotometric device that measures SpO_2 by determining the differential absorption of light by oxyhaemoglobin and deoxyhaemoglobin (Figure 10.2). Modern oximeters use a

---

ABC of COPD, 2nd edition.
Edited by Graeme P. Currie. © 2011 Blackwell Publishing Ltd.

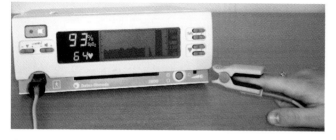

Figure 10.2 A pulse oximeter.

Table 10.1 Problems with pulse oximeters.

Clinical situation	Result
Jaundice/ hyperbilirubinaemia	Falsely low saturation
CO poisoning/high carboxyhaemoglobin	Falsely high saturation
Poor peripheral perfusion/hypothermia	Poor signal, unreliable
Nail varnish	Poor signal, unreliable

probe incorporating a light source and sensor that can be attached to the patient's finger or ear lobe. They are easy to use, portable, non-invasive and increasingly inexpensive. There is a short delay of 30 seconds in registration due to circulation time and they are less accurate at SpO_2 levels below 75%. Pulse oximeters should be available to assess all breathless or acutely ill patients in both primary and secondary care, although caution is required in interpretation in some circumstances (Table 10.1).

Oxygen during exacerbations of COPD

Some patients with advanced COPD (or during an exacerbation) have a fall in PaO_2 to <8 kPa and rise in $PaCO_2$; this is termed hypercapnic or type 2 respiratory failure. The mechanism underlying this problem is complex but it includes V/Q mismatching, reduced buffering capacity of haemoglobin, absorption atelectasis and reduced ventilatory drive. Providing high concentrations of oxygen in this situation can lead to diminished ventilation with further rise in $PaCO_2$ and development of respiratory acidosis, particularly if PaO_2 rises above 10 kPa. Indeed, many patients with COPD are 'acclimatised' to living with SpO_2 much lower than normal and are unlikely to benefit from a large increase even during an acute illness. In a large UK study of patients admitted to hospital with an exacerbation of COPD, as many as 47% had $PaCO_2$ >6.0 kPa, 20% had respiratory acidosis (pH <7.35) and 4.6% had severe acidosis (pH <7.25). Patients with severe COPD and previous episodes of hypercapnic respiratory failure during an exacerbation should therefore be given a personalised oxygen alert card to try and avoid administration of high concentrations of oxygen (Figure 10.3).

Prehospital oxygen

Prior to initiation of oxygen, patients should show their oxygen alert card to ambulance crew. A 28% Venturi mask at 4 l/min or 24% Venturi mask at 2 l/min, aiming for SpO_2 of 88–92%, should ideally be used in the community and during transport to hospital (Figures 10.4 and 10.5). The oxygen concentration should

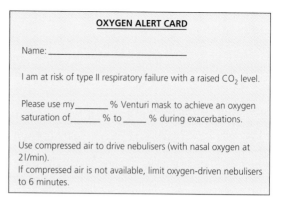

Figure 10.3 An example of an oxygen alert card.

OXYGEN ALERT CARD

Name: _____

I am at risk of type II respiratory failure with a raised CO_2 level.

Please use my _____ % Venturi mask to achieve an oxygen saturation of _____ % to _____ % during exacerbations.

Use compressed air to drive nebulisers (with nasal oxygen at 2 l/min).
If compressed air is not available, limit oxygen-driven nebulisers to 6 minutes.

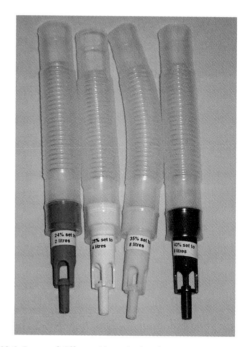

Figure 10.4 Range of different Venturi valves (24, 28, 35 and 40% are shown).

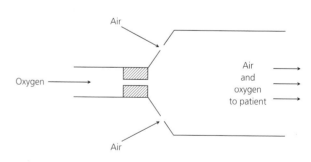

Figure 10.5 Mechanisms behind the Venturi system. Oxygen is delivered through the Venturi valve at a given flow rate; a fixed amount of air is entrapped and the inspired concentration of oxygen can be accurately predicted.

be reduced if SpO_2 exceeds 92% since this could lead to worsening CO_2 retention. If nebulised bronchodilators are administered, they should be given by compressed air and supplemental oxygen given through nasal cannulae at a flow rate of 2–4 l/min.

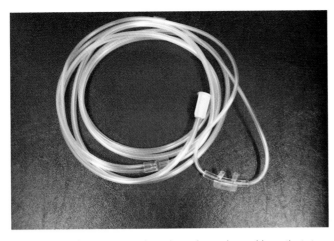

Figure 10.6 Delivering oxygen through nasal cannulae enables patients to eat, drink and communicate without difficulty.

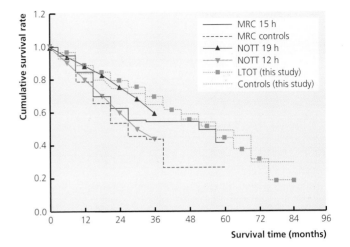

Figure 10.7 LTOT has been shown to prolong survival in patients with COPD when used for at least 15 hours/day. Figure reproduced with permission from Gorecka D, Gorzelak K, Sliwinski P, Tobiasz M, Zielinskiet J. *Thorax* 1997; **52**: 674–679.

Hospital oxygen

As soon as possible after arrival in hospital, an arterial blood gas measurement should be done. If pH and $PaCO_2$ are normal, aim for SpO_2 of 94–98% but if not, continue to aim for a target SpO_2 of 88–92%. Recheck arterial blood gases 30–60 minutes after starting oxygen (or altering its concentration) to confirm that $PaCO_2$ has not increased. Once patients are stabilised, consider changing from a Venturi mask to nasal cannulae at 1–2 l/min (Figure 10.6).

Long-term oxygen therapy

Two large randomised controlled trials have shown that using oxygen for at least 15 hours/day improves survival and quality of life in hypoxaemic patients with COPD (Figure 10.7). Long-term oxygen therapy (LTOT) should therefore be considered in non-smoking patients with COPD if

- $PaO_2 < 7.3$ kPa on two separate occasions at least 3 weeks apart during a period of clinical stability or,
- PaO_2 is between 7.3 and 8 kPa and there is evidence of secondary polycythaemia, pulmonary hypertension, peripheral oedema or nocturnal hypoxaemia.

Survival benefits have not been observed in patients with a PaO_2 of 7.3–8.0 kPa without secondary complications or those who do not use LTOT for a minimum of 15 hours each day. Before arranging LTOT, patients should ideally have stopped smoking and be made aware of the dangers of naked flames in the proximity of oxygen supplies. LTOT is most conveniently and economically given by a concentrator which removes nitrogen from the air and supplies oxygen-enriched air (Figure 10.8). Nasal cannulae are the most practical means of delivering LTOT, although some patients – especially those with troublesome dry nasal mucosa – may prefer a Venturi face mask.

Ambulatory oxygen

Ambulatory oxygen provides patients already receiving LTOT with portable oxygen during exercise and activities of daily living. This

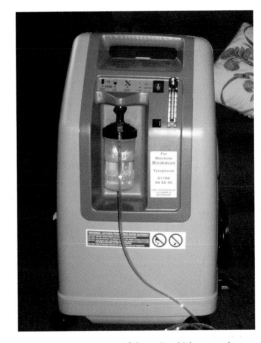

Figure 10.8 A concentrator is a useful way in which to supply oxygen to the patients without the need of cylinders. In Scotland, an oxygen concentrator can only be prescribed by a consultant chest physician.

should lead to greater patient independence and improved quality of life. However, its usefulness is currently limited by the duration of oxygen supply from portable-sized pulse dose cylinders. For example, a modern portable cylinder without an oxygen-conserving device will only last for up to 4 hours with a flow rate of 2 l/min and up to 2 hours with a flow rate of 4 l/min. Ambulatory oxygen therapy should also be considered in patients who have exercise desaturation, are shown to have an improvement in exercise capacity and/or breathlessness with oxygen and have the motivation to use oxygen.

Although liquid oxygen has been available in the United Kingdom for many years, it is only recently that this mode of supply has been used as a portable option for patients with COPD. Oxygen exists in a liquid state at temperatures below $-180\,^{\circ}$C and 30 l of liquid will provide 25,000 l of gas. There are specific risks associated with liquid oxygen including cold burns, leakage and problems with installation of a reservoir unit above ground floor level; liquid oxygen should only be prescribed after a risk assessment. A small portable flask can be filled quickly from the reservoir unit providing an instant source of ambulatory oxygen as and when required. Portable oxygen concentrators are also becoming available for specific situations which may, for example, permit patients to more easily go on holiday.

Continuous flow of oxygen via nasal cannulae or a mask is reliable but also very wasteful. About two-thirds of the supplied oxygen is wasted as the patient exhales. Oxygen-conserving devices, such as reservoir cannulae and demand pulsing devices, turn on the flow during inspiration and turn it off during expiration, leading to increased usage time and reduced cost of oxygen delivery.

Short burst oxygen

Despite maximal inhaled and oral pharmacological treatment, many patients with advanced COPD remain breathless on exertion. Oxygen delivered via cylinders is frequently prescribed for breathlessness at rest or during recovery after exercise. However, studies in patients who do not fulfil the arterial blood gas criteria for prescription of LTOT generally demonstrate that oxygen after exercise does not consistently influence breathlessness scores or rate of symptomatic recovery. Oxygen used in this way has been shown to reduce the degree of dynamic hyperinflation during recovery from exercise, but fails to significantly alter the degree of breathlessness. Whether there is actually a role for 'short burst' oxygen therapy in COPD is therefore controversial. Patients with episodes of severe breathlessness not relieved by other treatments should be thoroughly assessed including measurement of arterial blood gas tensions. Short burst oxygen should only be prescribed if clear improvement in breathlessness or exercise tolerance can be confirmed.

Air travel and oxygen

Increasing numbers of individuals at extremes of age and with a variety of medical problems such as COPD are travelling by air. Commercial aircraft fly at 27,000–37,000 feet (9,000–11,000 metres) and are required to maintain cabin pressure at the equivalent of 8,000 feet (2,438 m). At this pressure, inspired O_2 is

Table 10.2 Advice regarding necessity of in-flight oxygen in commercial aircraft.

Oxygen saturation on air	Recommendation
>95%	Oxygen not required
92–95% (without risk factor*)	Oxygen not required
92–95% (with risk factor*)	Hypoxic challenge test**
<92%	In-flight oxygen required (2 or 4 l/min)
Already receiving long-term oxygen therapy	Increase flow rate

*Risk factor: FEV_1 < 50% predicted, lung cancer, respiratory muscle weakness and other restrictive ventilatory disorders, within 6 weeks of hospital discharge.
**This involves subjects breathing 15% oxygen at sea level for 15–20 minutes to mimic the environment to which they would be exposed during a typical commercial flight. Those with pO_2 > 7.4 kPa post hypoxic challenge do not require in-flight oxygen, those with pO_2 < 6.6 kPa require in-flight oxygen and those with pO_2 6.6–7.4 kPa are considered borderline.

the equivalent of breathing 15% oxygen; even in healthy subjects, SpO_2 will fall. In patients with COPD, oxygenation may fall causing breathlessness and this desaturation will be exacerbated by minimal exercise.

For patients with moderate or severe COPD, SpO_2 should be measured on air using a pulse oximeter before flights are booked. Doing so helps determine whether in-flight oxygen is required or not (Table 10.2). All patients with COPD who require in-flight oxygen should inform the relevant airline when booking and be aware that some airlines charge for this service. The need for oxygen while changing flights must also be considered and many airports can provide wheelchairs for transport to and from aircraft. Patients should be advised to carry both preventative and reliever inhalers in hand luggage; nebulisers may be used at the discretion of the cabin crew.

Further reading

British Thoracic Society Standards of Care Committee. Managing passengers with respiratory disease planning air travel: British Thoracic Society recommendations. *Thorax* 2002; **57**: 289–304.

O'Driscoll BR, Howard LS, Davison AG. Guideline for emergency oxygen use in adult patients. *Thorax* 2008; **63**(suppl 6): vi1–vi68.

Plant PK, Owen JL, Elliot MW. One year period prevalence study of respiratory acidosis in acute exacerbations of COPD: implications for the provision of non-invasive ventilation and oxygen administration. *Thorax* 2000; **55**: 550–554.

Stevenson NS, Calverley PMA. Effect of oxygen on recovery from maximal exercise in patients with COPD. *Thorax* 2004; **59**: 668–672.

CHAPTER 11

Exacerbations

Graeme P. Currie[1] and Jadwiga A. Wedzicha[2]

[1]Aberdeen Royal Infirmary, Aberdeen, UK
[2]Royal Free and University College Medical School, University College, London, UK

OVERVIEW

- Exacerbations are important events in the natural history of chronic obstructive pulmonary disease (COPD) and are associated with a more rapid decline in lung function and health status
- Exacerbations of COPD should be treated promptly
- Inhaled bronchodilators form the mainstay of treatment
- A short course of oral corticosteroids should be given in most exacerbations affecting daily activities; antibiotics are most effective when there is a combination of increased breathlessness and increased sputum volume and purulence
- Non-invasive ventilation has revolutionised the management of hypercapnic exacerbations
- Aminophylline has a limited role in the management of exacerbations of COPD
- If admitted to hospital, strategies based around prevention of exacerbations should be explored

Definition

An exacerbation of chronic obstructive pulmonary disease (COPD) can be defined as a sustained worsening of respiratory symptoms that is acute in onset and usually requires a patient to seek medical help or alter medication. The deterioration must also be more severe than the usual variation experienced by the individual on a daily basis. From a pathophysiological perspective, exacerbations are associated with both local airway and systemic inflammation, which leads to further airflow obstruction, ventilation/perfusion mismatch and increased oxygen demands, pulmonary artery pressure and cardiac output. Exacerbations are characterised by a combination of increased

- breathlessness
- cough
- sputum volume
- sputum purulence
- wheeze
- chest tightness.

ABC of COPD, 2nd edition.
Edited by Graeme P. Currie. © 2011 Blackwell Publishing Ltd.

Other common clinical features include malaise, reduction in exercise tolerance, tachypnoea, tachycardia, peripheral oedema, accessory muscle use, confusion and cyanosis. Many other (and often coexisting) cardiorespiratory disorders can also cause some of these features and are included in the differential diagnosis (Box 11.1).

Box 11.1 **Differential diagnosis of an exacerbation of COPD**

- Exacerbation of asthma
- Bronchopneumonia
- Pulmonary embolism
- Pleural effusion
- Lung cancer
- Bronchiectasis
- Pneumothorax
- Upper airway obstruction
- Pulmonary oedema
- Cardiac arrhythmia e.g. atrial fibrillation

Aetiology

Exacerbations of COPD can be caused by viruses, bacteria, atypical organisms and environmental pollutants, although the exact cause remains unknown in many cases (Box 11.2). Viruses are thought to be implicated in causing around 50% of all exacerbations, with rhinoviruses and respiratory syncytial virus being some of the most commonly implicated. Viruses may also damage the airway epithelium and predispose to bacterial infection. It is uncertain how many exacerbations are caused by bacterial infection. However, bacteria can frequently be found in the sputum of clinically stable patients, and it is not clear whether exacerbations are caused by mutation of existing bacteria or the acquisition of new bacterial strains.

Box 11.2 **Causes of an exacerbation of COPD**

- Viruses
  - Rhinovirus
  - Respiratory syncytial virus
  - Influenza
  - Parainfluenza
  - Coronavirus
  - Adenovirus

- Bacteria
  - *Haemophilus influenzae*
  - *Streptococcus pneumoniae*
  - *Haemophilus parainfluenzae*
  - *Moraxella catarrhalis*
  - *Staphylococcus aurues*
  - *Pseudomonas aeruginosa*
  - Gram-negative bacilli
- Atypical organisms
  - *Chlamydia pneumoniae*
  - *Mycoplasma pneumoniae*
- Environmental pollutants
  - Ozone (O_3)
  - Sulphur dioxide (SO_2)
  - Nitrogen dioxide (NO_2)
  - Diesel exhaust fumes
  - Cigarette smoke

Impact

Exacerbations of COPD vary widely from mild episodes which can easily be managed at home to life-threatening events necessitating ventilatory support and a prolonged hospital stay. As a consequence, they have wide-reaching financial implications for secondary care providers and are likely to be partly responsible for high hospital bed occupancy rates. With the ever-increasing aged population, it is likely that the numbers of exacerbations treated both in the community and within hospitals will continue to rise. A report by the British Lung foundation (Invisible Lives) has identified areas within the United Kingdom where individuals are at highest risk of hospital admission because of COPD (Figure 11.1). Data relating to inpatient mortality from COPD is variable, with estimates ranging between 4% and 30%; the vast majority of acute episodes treated within the community do not result in death.

Patients with a history of frequent exacerbations have an accelerated decline in lung function and health status, impaired quality

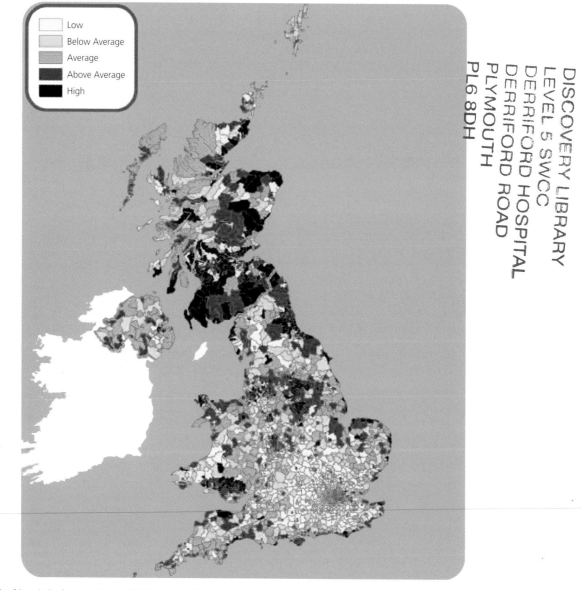

Figure 11.1 The risk of hospital admission due to COPD in the United Kingdom. Reproduced with permission from the British Lung Foundation. Copyright © 2005 Experian Ltd. Mapping: Copyright © 2006 Navteq.

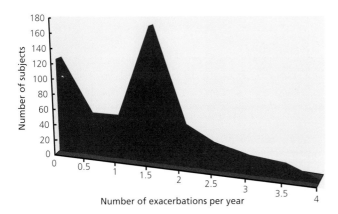

Figure 11.2 The non-normal distribution of exacerbations of COPD within a population. Reproduced with permission from S Scott, P Walker, PMA Calverley. COPD exacerbations: prevention. *Thorax* 2006; **61**: 440–447.

of life and restriction of daily living activities. This in turn increases the likelihood of a patient becoming housebound. Individuals with more advanced disease usually experience more exacerbations, although there is fairly wide inter-individual variation (Figure 11.2). Moreover, some appear susceptible to a greater exacerbation frequency and more rapid decline in lung function than others.

Investigations

If admitted to hospital, patients should be investigated as shown in Box 11.3.

Box 11.3 **Investigations required in patients admitted to hospital**

- Full blood count
- Biochemistry and glucose
- Theophylline concentration (in patients using a theophylline preparation)
- Arterial blood gas (documenting the amount of oxygen given and by what delivery device)
- Electrocardiograph
- Chest X-ray
- Blood cultures in febrile patients
- Sputum microscopy, culture and sensitivity

Management

Oxygen

Administration of oxygen is vital in all patients with respiratory failure to reduce breathlessness and prevent major organ and tissue hypoxaemia (see Chapter 10 for a more detailed description). In patients with type 2 respiratory failure (Table 11.1), controlled oxygen (24% or 28%) through a Venturi system should be given to keep the oxygen saturation between 88–92%. In individuals with type 1 respiratory failure, the oxygen concentration should be titrated upwards to achieve a target saturation range of 94–98%. After giving oxygen for $1/2$–1 hour, arterial blood gas levels should be rechecked – especially in those with type 2 respiratory failure. This allows the detection of a rise in carbon dioxide level or

Table 11.1 Arterial blood gas features of type 1 and type 2 respiratory failure.

	Type 1 respiratory failure	Type 2 respiratory failure
pO_2	↓	↓
pCO_2	↔ or ↓	↑
HCO_3	↔	↑ or ↔
pH	↔ or ↑	↔ or ↓

↑, increase; ↓, decrease; ↔, no change.

fall in pH due to loss of hypoxic drive. Deteriorating oxygen saturation or increasing breathlessness in a patient with previously stable hypoxaemia should also prompt repeat arterial blood gas measurements.

Bronchodilators

Short-acting bronchodilators (β2-agonists and anticholinergics) form the mainstay of treatment in exacerbations as they reduce symptoms and improve lung function. β2-agonists (such as salbutamol) increase the concentrations of cyclic adenosine monophosphate (cAMP) and stimulate β2-adrenoceptors, producing smooth muscle relaxation and bronchodilation, while anticholinergics (such as ipratropium) exert their bronchodilator effects predominantly by inhibition at muscarinic receptors. Salbutamol has an onset of action within 5 minutes and peaks at around 30 minutes, while ipratropium takes effect at 10–15 minutes and has a peak effect between 30 and 60 minutes; the duration of action of both is 4–6 hours. Although there are few data supporting any additional benefit in acute exacerbations, both classes of short-acting bronchodilators may be used together.

Short-acting bronchodilators can successfully be given by a metered dose inhaler plus spacer or nebuliser with similar efficacy. However, nebulisers (with a mouth or face mask) are independent of patient effort and are often more convenient than hand-held devices in the accident and emergency department or busy ward setting (Figure 11.3). In patients with hypercapnia or respiratory acidosis, nebulised bronchodilators should usually be driven by compressed air and supplemental oxygen given via a nasal cannula.

Corticosteroids

Over the years, studies have generally shown that systemic corticosteroids are of benefit in exacerbations of COPD. In particular, when compared to placebo, they improve lung function more rapidly, reduce the length of hospital stay and chance of treatment failure, and improve symptoms (Figure 11.4). The mechanism by which they exert their effects is uncertain, although may attenuate both local and systemic inflammatory processes. In the absence of major contraindications, oral corticosteroids should therefore be given to all patients with an exacerbation of COPD. In severely ill patients or in those who are unable to swallow, 100–200 mg of intravenous hydrocortisone 8–12 hourly is a suitable alternative. In straightforward exacerbations, current guidelines recommend that 30–40 mg of prednisolone should be given for between 7 and 14 days; little further benefit is found in longer dosing regimes. In patients using oral corticosteroids for <3 weeks, it is not usually necessary to taper the dose downwards before discontinuation.

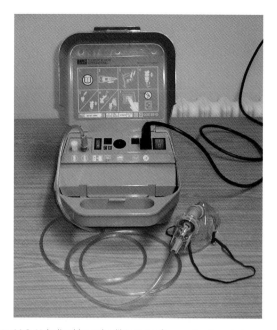

Figure 11.3 Nebulised bronchodilators are frequently given during an exacerbation of COPD.

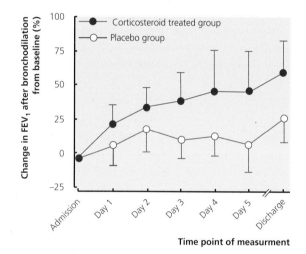

Time point of measurment

Figure 11.4 Difference in forced expiratory volume in 1 second (FEV₁) with oral corticosteroids compared to placebo in patients admitted with an exacerbation of COPD. Figure reproduced with permission from Davies *et al.* Oral corticosteroids in patients admitted to hospital with exacerbations of chronic obstructive pulmonary disease: a prospective randomised controlled trial. *Lancet* 1999; **354**: 456–460.

Antibiotics

Individuals with COPD have relatively high concentrations of bacteria in their airways during both exacerbations and periods of clinical stability, although the overall benefits of antibiotics remain contentious. Moreover, injudicious antibiotic use may be implicated in the emergence of resistant strains of bacteria and enteric infections such as *Clostridium difficile*, while many exacerbations are caused by viruses and pollutants. Guidelines suggest that antibiotics are most effective when patients have more severe exacerbations characterised by increased breathlessness, sputum

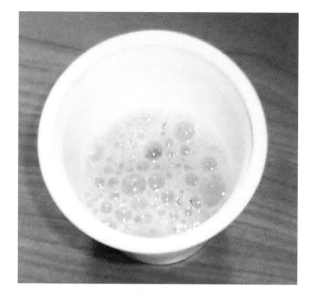

Figure 11.5 Antibiotics are most effective when patients have a combination of increased breathlessness, and increased sputum volume and purulence.

volume and purulence (Figure 11.5). The oral route is preferred unless the patient is vomiting, severely unwell or unable to swallow. The choice of antibiotic should be tailored to local sensitivities; amoxycillin (or clarithromycin in penicillin-allergic patients) is a reasonable first choice in those with mild to moderate COPD, while anti-pseudomonal antibiotics (such as ciprofloxacin) should be considered in those with advanced disease.

Aminophylline

Aminophylline has historically been used in exacerbations of COPD, despite a paucity of data demonstrating any major benefit. When compared to placebo, aminophylline has only limited (if any) effect upon symptoms, lung function and length of hospital stay in non-acidotic patients. Moreover, its use is associated with adverse effects such as nausea, vomiting and tachyarrythmias. The routine addition of aminophylline in most exacerbations of COPD is therefore not warranted. Increasing evidence suggests that even at low doses, theophylline activates histone deacetylases (thereby attenuating the effects of activated pro-inflammatory mechanisms), although within the context of an exacerbation, the significance of this is unknown.

Current guidelines do suggest the addition of aminophylline to standard therapy in patients with moderate-to-severe exacerbations or those not responding to nebulised bronchodilators and other treatments. In patients not using an oral theophylline preparation, a loading dose of 5 mg/kg over at least 20 minutes with cardiac monitoring should be given with subsequent maintenance infusion of 0.5 mg/kg/hour. In patients already using a theophylline preparation, the loading dose should be omitted and a plasma level ideally obtained prior to commencement of a maintenance infusion of 0.5 mg/kg/hour. Daily plasma theophylline levels should be measured and the infusion rate altered to maintain a concentration of between 10 and 20 mg/l (55–110 μmol/l).

Respiratory stimulants

Since the introduction of non-invasive ventilation (NIV), the use of doxapram has become far less common in hypercapnic respiratory failure. It may have some use in patients in whom NIV is contraindicated or when NIV is not immediately available. Whether doxapram confers benefit when used alongside NIV is uncertain. Doxapram is given by continuous intravenous infusion and stimulates both respiratory and non-respiratory muscles. Its use is often limited by adverse effects such as agitation, tachycardia, confusion and hallucinations.

Non-invasive ventilation

NIV has revolutionised the management of hypercapnic respiratory failure due to COPD and is comprehensively discussed in Chapter 12.

General hospital care

Measures to prevent venous thromboembolism with low molecular weight heparin should be considered in all patents admitted with an exacerbation of COPD. Attention should also be given to adequate hydration and nutritional input. Many patients also have important co-morbidities – for example, ischaemic heart disease, left ventricular dysfunction and diabetes mellitus – which must not be overlooked. Early pulmonary rehabilitation and physiotherapy as soon after an exacerbation as possible should be encouraged, as improvements in exercise capacity and overall heath status may occur. When recovering from an exacerbation in hospital, it is useful for many patients to be reviewed by physiotherapists and occupational therapists. Physiotherapists may be able to provide advice on breathlessness, panic and anxiety management, energy conservation techniques and walking aids, while occupational therapists can offer practical solutions in daily living activities.

Intravenous magnesium is advocated in exacerbations of asthma, but is of no known benefit in COPD. It should therefore not be given.

Assisted hospital discharge

Any intervention which successfully hastens a patient's recovery and discharge from hospital can be seen to be potentially useful in the overall management of an exacerbation. In recent years, 'assisted hospital discharge' or 'hospital at home' schemes have been developed, whereby patients with non-severe exacerbations can be relatively immediately discharged back into the community (after initial assessment in hospital) with appropriate nursing and medical back up. Apart from providing patients with a package of care, this practice also facilitates the identification of a deterioration in clinical condition and readmission to hospital if necessary. Studies have shown that hospital readmission and mortality rates are not significantly different when assisted discharge schemes have been compared to standard inpatient care. Moreover, such schemes may lead to financial savings along with increased availability of inpatient beds. Not all patients admitted with an exacerbation of COPD are suitable for assisted discharge, and relative contraindications are highlighted in Box 11.4.

Box 11.4 **Relative contraindications to assisted hospital discharge in patients with an exacerbation of COPD**

- Acute onset
- Confusion
- Worsening peripheral oedema
- Uncertain diagnosis
- Poor performance status
- Concomitant unstable medical disorders
- New chest X-ray abnormalities
- Acidosis or marked hypoxia or hypercapnia
- Adverse social conditions

Monitoring while in hospital

Clinical assessment and routine observations are useful in assessing the rate of recovery from an exacerbation. Frequent arterial blood gas measurements are also required to monitor patients with decompensated respiratory acidosis. Daily recordings of peak expiratory flow rates are less useful, unless the patient has reversible obstructive lung disease. It is useful to record spirometry prior to discharge as this helps confirm the diagnosis (in patients who have not previously had it performed), provides information regarding the severity of airflow obstruction and enables progress to be assessed at subsequent outpatient follow-up.

Outpatient follow-up

Early follow-up (e.g. within 3 weeks) either in the community or secondary care should be arranged following hospital discharge as this may help prevent readmission. This facilitates an opportunity to explore strategies to prevent a further exacerbation and provide education, check inhaler technique, alter inhaled treatment if required, check oxygen saturation and arterial blood gases where necessary and reassess smoking status.

It should also be made clear to patients that exacerbations should be promptly treated in the future; doing so results in a quicker recovery than if a delay is encountered. Moreover, patients who frequently fail to promptly report or recognise worsening symptoms have a greater risk of being admitted to hospital and generally have a poorer quality of life.

Frequent exacerbations

It is well established that many patients with COPD have frequent exacerbations necessitating repeated hospital admissions. This is especially the case in individuals with hypercapnic respiratory failure who have had treatment with NIV. Indeed, within a year after hospital discharge, it is likely that the majority of these patients will be readmitted to hospital and require further NIV, with as many as half dying. Further studies are required to identify factors associated with readmission and devise ways by which to address this common problem.

Prevention of exacerbations

Many non-pharmacological and pharmacological strategies have been shown to reduce the frequency of exacerbations of COPD. Examples of these include early pulmonary rehabilitation, lung volume reduction surgery, long-term oxygen, long-acting bronchodilators, inhaled corticosteroids and mucolytics, details of which are discussed in separate chapters.

Further reading

Barr RG, Rowe BH, Camargo CA Jr. Methylxanthines for exacerbations of chronic obstructive pulmonary disease. *The Cochrane Database of Systematic Reviews* 2003; (2). Art. No.: CD002168. DOI: 10.1002/14651858.CD002168.

Chu CM, Chan VL, Lin AWN, Wong IWY, Leung WS, Lai CKW. Readmission rates and life-threatening events in COPD survivors treated with non-invasive ventilation for hypercapnic respiratory failure. *Thorax* 2004; **59**: 1020–1025.

Man WD, Polkey MI, Donaldson N, Gray BJ, Moxham J. Community pulmonary rehabilitation after hospitalisation for acute exacerbations of chronic obstructive pulmonary disease: randomised controlled study. *BMJ* 2004; **329**: 1209.

McCrory DC, Brown CD. Anticholinergic bronchodilators versus beta2-sympathomimetic agents for acute exacerbations of chronic obstructive pulmonary disease. *The Cochrane Database of Systematic Reviews* 2002, (3). Art. No.: CD003900. DOI: 10.1002/14651858.CD003900.

Rodríguez-Roisin R. COPD exacerbations: management. *Thorax* 2006; **61**: 535–544.

Seemungal TA, Donaldson GC, Bhowmik A, Jeffries DJ, Wedzicha JA. Time course and recovery of exacerbations in patients with chronic obstructive pulmonary disease. *American Journal of Respiratory and Critical Care Medicine* 2000; **161**: 1608–1613.

Wilkinson TMA, Donaldson GC, Hurst JR, Seemungal TAR, Wedzicha JA. Early therapy improves outcomes of exacerbations of chronic obstructive pulmonary disease. *American Journal of Respiratory and Critical Care Medicine* 2004; **168**: 1298–1303.

Wood-Baker RR, Gibson PG, Hannay M, Walters EH, Walters JAE. Systemic corticosteroids for acute exacerbations of chronic obstructive pulmonary disease. *The Cochrane Database of Systematic Reviews* 2005, (1). Art. No.: CD001288.pub2. DOI: 10.1002/14651858.CD001288.pub2.

CHAPTER 12

Non-invasive Ventilation

Paul K. Plant[1] *and Graeme P. Currie*[2]

[1]St James's University Hospital, Leeds, UK
[2]Aberdeen Royal Infirmary, Aberdeen, UK

OVERVIEW

In exacerbations of chronic obstructive pulmonary disease (COPD):

- Non-invasive ventilation (NIV) reduces mortality and the need for intubation in patients with a respiratory acidosis (pH < 7.35 and $PaCO_2$ > 6 kPa)

- NIV should be considered within the first 60 minutes of hospital arrival in all patients in whom a respiratory acidosis persists despite maximum medical therapy

- NIV should be initiated only by trained staff; monitoring should include respiratory rate, arterial blood gases, pulse oximetry, synchrony and compliance

- NIV should be continued until the underlying acute cause has resolved

- All patients should have a clear plan recorded and agreed upon in the event of NIV failure

---

Non-invasive ventilation (NIV) has revolutionised the management and survival of patients with an acidotic exacerbation of chronic obstructive pulmonary disease (COPD). Indeed, it is difficult to justify admitting patients with an exacerbation of COPD to hospitals where no relatively immediate facility to provide NIV is available. A close fitting face or nose mask connected to a portable ventilator by tubing facilitates a non-invasive method of providing respiratory support (mechanically assisted or mechanically generated breaths) to the spontaneously breathing patient (Figure 12.1). The mask can be easily removed, which in turn allows patients to communicate, eat, drink, undergo physiotherapy and receive nebulised and oral medication more easily than other forms of ventilation. NIV provides many other advantages over invasive mechanical ventilation (Box 12.1).

How non-invasive ventilation works

NIV provides a bi-level form of respiratory support. Ventilation is provided by inspiratory positive airways pressure (IPAP), which is usually titrated from 10 to between 15 and 20 cmH_2O. This

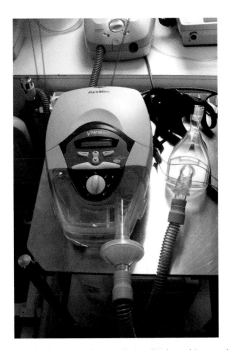

Figure 12.1 A typical non-invasive ventilation (NIV) machine can be easily used at the patient's bedside.

helps to offload tiring respiratory muscles and reduce the work of breathing, improve alveolar ventilation and oxygenation and increase CO_2 elimination.

Box 12.1 **Advantages of NIV over invasive mechanical ventilation**

- Patients can eat and drink.
- Patients can communicate and make decisions about management.
- Patients maintain a physiological cough.
- Physiological warming and humidification occurs.
- No sedatives required.
- Reduced risk of ventilator-associated pneumonia.
- Less expensive and intensive care bed is not necessarily required.
- Allows intermittent use, which facilitates weaning.
- Endotracheal intubation remains an option.

ABC of COPD, 2nd edition.
Edited by Graeme P. Currie. © 2011 Blackwell Publishing Ltd.

During expiration, the expiratory positive airways pressure (EPAP) helps 'splint open' the airway and flushes CO_2 from the mask. It also reduces the work of breathing by overcoming intrinsic positive end expiratory pressure, thereby reducing atelectasis and increasing end tidal volume; usual pressures are between 4 and 6 cmH_2O. Oxygen is usually introduced either through a port in the face mask or through a channel found more proximally in the ventilator system. The exact fraction of inspired oxygen delivered to the patient is usually unknown and oxygen entrainment should be titrated against pulse oximetry. Humidification is rarely required.

When to use non-invasive ventilation in COPD

NIV should be considered within the first 60 minutes of hospital arrival in all patients with an acute exacerbation of COPD in whom a respiratory acidosis (pH < 7.35 and pCO_2 > 6 kPa) persists despite maximum medical therapy. This includes nebulised bronchodilators, steroids, antibiotics (where indicated) and controlled oxygen to maintain SpO_2 at 88–92% (Chapter 11). NIV can also be used as a therapeutic trial prior to proceeding to mechanical ventilation, or when more invasive ventilatory support is inappropriate. In the latter circumstance, NIV is therefore considered the 'ceiling of treatment'.

Many studies with differing endpoints – such as mortality, need for intubation, arterial blood gas values and cost-effectiveness – have consistently shown significant benefits with NIV over and above conventional medical treatment alone. For example, a meta-analysis of eight randomised controlled trials evaluated effects of NIV in patients admitted with an exacerbation of COPD with pCO_2 > 6 kPa. This study demonstrated that compared to standard treatment alone, the use of concomitant NIV was associated with:

- lower mortality
- reduced need for intubation
- reduced likelihood of treatment failure
- a lower complication rate
- improvements at 1 hour in pH, pCO_2 and respiratory rate
- a shorter stay in hospital.

Setting

NIV can be successfully used in the ward setting and in high dependency and intensive care units. It can also be commenced in accident and emergency departments, although in many cases, patients will not have had sufficient time to respond to conventional treatment. The exact setting is less important, provided there are suitably trained nurses, physiotherapists and medical staff available to initiate treatment, monitor progress and troubleshoot. For patients with COPD, there is little to guide ventilator selection other than familiarity, cost and local preference. If NIV is used for hypoxic respiratory failure, the ventilator unit needs an intrinsic blender to ensure that high fractions of inspired oxygen can be delivered. Intensive care ventilators are often difficult to use non-invasively as they are 'poorly leak tolerant' and alarm readily.

How to use non-invasive ventilation

Prior to starting NIV, it should be decided and documented whether the patient is a suitable candidate for invasive mechanical ventilation or whether relative contraindications to NIV exist (Box 12.2). Caution is advised in commencing NIV in moribund patients in whom intubation (at one end of the extreme) or a palliative approach (at the other end) might be a more appropriate and pragmatic strategy. The views of the patient and family as to whether they would wish further respiratory support if NIV proves unsuccessful should also be taken into account. Any escalation plan (or otherwise) should be clearly documented within the medical and nursing notes.

> **Box 12.2 Relative contraindications to NIV; none of these are absolute and the clinical context needs to be considered**
>
> - Confusion/agitation
> - Inability to maintain airway
> - Reduced Glasgow Coma Scale
> - Haemodynamic instability
> - Vomiting
> - Copious respiratory secretions and risk of aspiration
> - Facial burns/surgery/trauma
> - Severe hypoxia
> - Untreated pneumothorax
> - Severe pneumonia/sepsis
> - Fixed upper airway obstruction
> - Bowel obstruction
> - Bronchopleural fistula

Provided the clinical condition permits, the patient should be shown the ventilator, face mask and tubing; an appropriately sized face mask (sizing rings are usually provided by the manufacturer) should then be chosen (Figure 12.2). Nasal masks may also be used and are comfortable for long-term use, but require the patient to breathe through their nose. However, most patients with acute exacerbations of COPD breathe through their mouth and full face

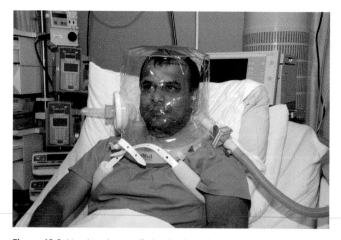

Figure 12.2 Non-invasive ventilation (NIV) can be given using a full face or nose mask, which come in a variety of sizes; a hood (shown above) can be used in patients intolerant of these options.

masks are therefore preferable. It is useful if the face mask is first placed on the patient for several minutes prior to securing it with straps. The oxygen should be set an initial appropriate flow rate (typically 1–2 l/min) and adjusted to maintain a saturation between 88% and 92%.

The IPAP and EPAP should be set at fairly low pressures such as 10 cmH$_2$O and 4 cmH$_2$O respectively. The inspiratory pressure can then be titrated up in 2–5 cmH$_2$O increments to 15–20 cmH$_2$O or to the maximum pressure comfortably tolerated. Depending on the type of ventilator, other parameters such as the sensitivity of the inspiratory and expiratory triggers and maximum inspiratory and expiratory times may be set. Adjustments to these may be necessary to maximise synchrony between the ventilator and the efforts of the patient. Once started, patient comfort, breathing synchrony and compliance are key factors for success with NIV. In some individuals with shallow breathing or low respiratory rates, it may be necessary to programme the NIV machine to deliver a minimum number of breaths per minute.

Monitoring non-invasive ventilation

Irrespective of pO$_2$ or pCO$_2$, the pH is a reliable marker of severity in exacerbations of COPD, and is closely linked to mortality and the need for intubation. In addition to regular recording of pulse, blood pressure and respiratory rate, the oxygen saturation should be monitored and number of hours of NIV use documented. Arterial blood gases should be checked 1 hour after starting NIV; an improvement in pH, pCO$_2$ and reduction in respiratory rate are good prognostic signs. If no improvement occurs, the mask should be checked for leaks, all tubing and connections checked for problems, the ventilator checked for synchrony with the patient's respiratory effort and consideration given to adjusting the ventilator settings (e.g. IPAP or oxygen flow rate). Blood gases should be rechecked 4–6 hours after NIV initiation (or earlier in the event of a clinical deterioration) and within an hour of a change in ventilator setting (Figure 12.3).

NIV should be continued until the underlying acute cause resolves, typically for 3–4 days, although sometimes only 24 hours of treatment is required. However, NIV should not be discontinued as soon as the pH first normalises. Weaning from NIV is rarely a problem, as patients normally 'auto wean' by progressively decreasing their use automatically (e.g. by way of progressively longer 'NIV-free' periods initially throughout the day and later at night).

Other measures

Maximal medical therapy such as nebulised bronchodilators, corticosteroids and antibiotics in patients commenced on NIV should be continued. Patients should avoid sedative drugs such as benzodiazepines and opiates, which may require pharmacological reversal, especially if the respiratory rate is low. Patients should be kept adequately hydrated and an adequate calorific intake maintained (Figure 12.4). Nebulised bronchodilators should be given during 'NIV-free' periods when possible, as NIV impairs aerosol formation and lung delivery.

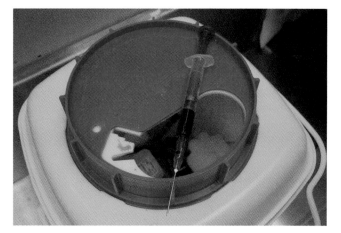

Figure 12.3 Frequent monitoring of arterial blood gases is required in patients using non-invasive ventilation (NIV). These should be performed prior to starting NIV and 1 and 4–6 hours afterwards; they should also be checked within an hour of changing settings.

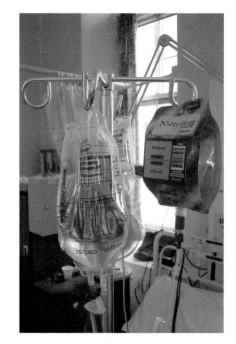

Figure 12.4 Patients being treated with non-invasive ventilation (NIV) can easily become dehydrated and undernourished; adequate hydration and nutrition should not be forgotten in overall management.

Problems with non-invasive ventilation

The majority of patients tolerate NIV without significant problems. However, some patients experience difficulty in 'breathing with the machine'. The mask can be associated with problems such as claustrophobia, facial sores and persistent air leaks (Figure 12.5). Box 12.3 provides guidance on managing common problems. Patients who recover from an exacerbation treated with NIV are at high risk of a future exacerbation requiring NIV, and should be asked whether they would wish ventilatory support in the future.

Box 12.3 **Problems associated with NIV and potential solutions**

Problem	Possible solutions
Persistent hypoxia	Re-evaluate patient and optimise medical treatment
	Check compliance with ventilation and synchrony
	Check head position/airway
	Exclude pneumothorax
	Check oxygen tubing for leaks/blockages
	Increase oxygen flow rate
	Increase IPAP to a maximum of 25 cmH$_2$O
	Increase EPAP by small amounts
	Arrange intubation and ventilation
	Consider palliation (if NIV is the 'ceiling of treatment')
Persisting hypercapnia/ respiratory acidosis	Re-evaluate patient and optimise medical treatment
	Check compliance with ventilation and synchrony
	Check head position/airway
	Exclude pneumothorax
	Avoid sedating drugs
	Increase IPAP to a maximum of 25 cmH$_2$O
	Reduce oxygen flow if saturation >88–92%
	Increase back-up rate if respiratory rate low
	Ensure expiratory port is patent
	Arrange intubation and ventilation
	Consider palliation (if NIV is the 'ceiling of treatment')
Respiratory alkalosis/ hypocapnia	Reduce IPAP
	Reduce back-up respiratory rate
	Reduce hours of use
	Ensure serum potassium >4 mmol/l
Nasal/forehead ulceration	Loosen straps
	Apply dressing
	Longer 'rest periods' without NIV
	Consider full head mask/nasal plugs
Nasal congestion	Nasally inhaled corticosteroids
	Nasally inhaled decongestants (short-term use only)
	Change nasal mask to full face mask
	Humidification
Mask leak	Readjust straps and mask (may paradoxically require loosening)
	Change to a more suitably sized face mask
Claustrophobia	Consider different mask (nasal or full head mask)
	Allow patient to hold the mask in position
NIV dependence	More gradual discontinuation
	Distracting techniques while not using NIV
	Reassurance
Gastric distension	Reduce IPAP
	Reduce EPAP
	Insert a fine-bore nasogastric tube
Confusion/ delirium	Monitor in high dependency setting
	Minimise procedures and contacts
	Correct oxygen and carbon dioxide as soon as possible
	Consider other causes of confusion (such as alcohol withdrawal)
	Consider sedative drugs (e.g. haloperidol) if persistently aggressive or agitated

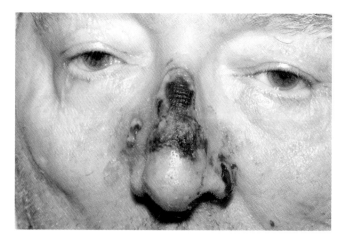

Figure 12.5 Severe nasal bridge ulceration in a patient who required non-invasive ventilation (NIV) for a prolonged period of time. Figure reproduced with permission from Dr David Miller, Aberdeen Royal Infirmary, Aberdeen.

Domiciliary non-invasive ventilation

The role of domiciliary NIV in COPD is controversial. Unlike patients with neuromuscular disorders, compliance tends to be poorer once at home. Randomised controlled trials have failed to show either a definite survival advantage or quality of life improvement. However, in hypoxic patients with COPD who develop hypercapnia or acidosis while receiving long-term oxygen therapy, domiciliary nocturnal NIV may be useful. Domiciliary NIV can also be useful in patients with hypercapnic respiratory failure who are frequently admitted to hospital with exacerbations associated with development of an acidosis.

Mechanical ventilation

Invasive mechanical ventilation should be considered in patients established on NIV whose pH, pCO$_2$ and respiratory rate have

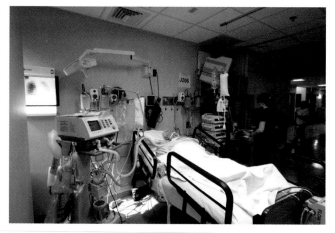

Figure 12.6 Not all patients with an exacerbation of COPD are suitable candidates for invasive mechanical ventilation as successful outcome is unlikely in some; factors such as co-morbidities, body mass index and nutritional status, premorbid functional status, lung function, age, and patient and family wishes should all be taken into account. Figure reproduced from sciencephoto.com.

deteriorated or failed to improve within 4–6 hours of initiation (Figure 12.6); in such patients, it is less likely that NIV will be successful. In those with more severe acidosis – such as an initial pH < 7.26 – it is also less likely that NIV will result in a favourable outcome but a therapeutic trial may still be appropriate, ideally in a high dependency or intensive care setting. Other situations favouring the use of invasive mechanical ventilation over NIV include severe hypoxia, severe breathlessness, severe tachypnoea and paradoxical abdominal movement, inability to tolerate NIV, respiratory arrest, pneumonia, severe sepsis, cardiovascular instability and pulmonary embolism. Individuals who initially improve but become acidotic again after 48 hours tend to have a poor prognosis and higher mortality rate if NIV is continued than if mechanical ventilation is initiated. The latter treatment option should therefore be considered.

The long-term survival of patients with COPD who require mechanical ventilation is generally poorer compared to those who require NIV alone. However, failure of NIV should not be used as a reason to decline invasive mechanical ventilation and does not imply that these patients will be difficult to wean. In patients receiving invasive mechanical ventilation, NIV has an important role in weaning. In other patients who cannot be weaned onto NIV within 48–72 hours of initiation, early percutaneous tracheostomy fashioning may facilitate weaning and help reduce the time spent in intensive care.

Further reading

British Thoracic Society Standards of Care Committee. Non-invasive ventilation in acute respiratory failure. *Thorax* 2002; **57**: 192–211.

Brochard L. Mechanical ventilation: invasive versus non-invasive. *European Respiratory Journal 2003*: **22**: 31s–37s.

Chu CM, Chan VL, Lin AWN, Wong IWY, Leung WS, Lai CKW. Readmission rates and life-threatening events in COPD survivors treated with non-invasive ventilation for acute hypercapnic respiratory failure. *Thorax* 2004; **59**: 1020–1025.

Lightowler JV, Wedzicha JA, Elliott, MW, Ram FSF. Non-invasive positive pressure ventilation to treat respiratory failure resulting from exacerbations of chronic obstructive pulmonary disease: Cochrane systematic review and meta-analysis. *BMJ* 2003; **326**: 185–190.

McLaughlin K, Thain G, Murray I, Currie GP. Ward based non-invasive ventilation for exacerbations of COPD: a real-life perspective. *Quarterly Journal of Medicine* 2010; **103**: 505–510.

Plant PK, Owen JL, Elliott MW. One year period prevalence study of respiratory acidosis in acute exacerbations of COPD: implications for the provision of non-invasive ventilation and oxygen administration. *Thorax* 2000; **55**: 550–554.

Plant PK, Owen JL, Elliott MW. Non-invasive ventilation in acute exacerbations of chronic obstructive pulmonary disease: long-term survival and predictors of in-hospital outcome. *Thorax* 2001; **56**: 708–712.

Quon B S, Gan W Q, Sin D D. Contemporary management of acute exacerbations of COPD: a systematic review and meta-analysis. *Chest* 2008; **133**: 756–766.

CHAPTER 13

Primary Care

Cathy Jackson

Bute Medical School, University of St Andrews, St Andrews, UK

OVERVIEW

- COPD is usually diagnosed and managed solely in primary care
- The UK Quality Outcome Framework defines a set of clinical indicators which should guide primary care health teams
- Primary care teams should maintain a high index of suspicion that COPD is present in all patients over 35 years who have a history of smoking

Over the past few decades, it has become increasingly apparent that chronic obstructive pulmonary disease (COPD) can place an enormous burden upon patients, families, healthcare systems, communities and society at large. General practitioners (GPs) are ideally placed to diagnose COPD and orchestrate its subsequent non-pharmacological and pharmacological management, most of which can take place almost entirely within a community setting. For many patients, community multidisciplinary team members also play an important role in overall management, although specialist secondary care assistance is required in certain circumstances.

The Quality Outcomes Framework (QOF) of the UK GP contract has recognised the importance of good management of COPD in primary care; this defines a set of clinical indicators based on current best available evidence. These indices look at the diagnosis and monitoring of disease, together with provision of strategies to prevent disease progression and acute exacerbations. Most GPs and primary healthcare teams have been implementing many of the recommendations for some time and they already realise the importance of a means of identifying patients with COPD, a good recording system for all data relating to care and a management framework.

Identification of patients

When faced with a patient who may have COPD, it is important to arrive at an accurate diagnosis and exclude alternative or concomitant conditions (Chapter 3). The primary healthcare team is well placed to do this, often having knowledge of a patient's previous

ABC of COPD, 2nd edition.
Edited by Graeme P. Currie. © 2011 Blackwell Publishing Ltd.

medical history both for major events and more trivial episodes such as recurrent chest infections, chronic cough and breathlessness. The diagnosis of COPD is fully described in Chapters 3 and 4 and relies upon a consistent history, examination findings and spirometric evidence of airflow obstruction.

COPD should be considered a treatable disease and improvements in long-term health status and mortality are possible if it is identified early and optimally managed. For this reason, GPs should maintain a high index of suspicion when presented with any patient with any relevant respiratory symptom who currently smokes (or with a history of cigarette smoking). Where resources allow, those who smoke cigarettes (or have a smoking history) and who are >35 years of age should be screened for COPD using a health questionnaire (Tables 13.1 and 13.2). Early diagnosis allows early intervention and may help reinforce the potential health gains to be achieved if a patient were to stop smoking.

Once a diagnosis of COPD has been made it is helpful to keep an accurate record of patients details and ensure optimal follow-up and management. The General Medical Services (GMS) quality

Table 13.1 A simple questionnaire for evaluating risk of COPD.

Patient characteristic	Value	Score*
Age (years)?	40–49	0
	50–59	4
	60–69	8
	≥70	10
Smoking pack years?	0–14	0
	15–24	2
	25–49	3
	≥50	7
Body mass index?	<25.4	5
	25.4–29.7	1
	>29.7	0
Cough affected by weather?	Yes	3
	No or no cough	0
Sputum production in absence of a cold?	Yes	3
	No	0
Sputum production first thing in the morning?	Yes	0
	No	3
Wheezes?	Sometimes or often	4
	Never	0
Has or used to have any allergies?	Yes	0
	No	3

*Total scores of ≥17 suggest increased risk of COPD being present.

Table 13.2 A simple questionnaire for differential diagnosis of COPD.

Patient characteristic	Value	Score*
Age (years)?	40–49	0
	50–59	5
	60–69	9
	≥70	11
Smoking pack years?	0–14	0
	15–24	3
	25–49	7
	≥50	9
Increased frequency of cough in recent years?	Yes	0
	No	1
Breathing problems in past 3 years?†	Yes	0
	No	3
Ever admitted to hospital with breathing problems?	Yes	6
	No	0
Short of breath more often in recent years?	Yes	1
	No	0
How much sputum coughed up most days?	<15 ml/day	0
	≥15 ml/day	4
When gets a cold it usually goes to chest?	Yes	4
	No	0
Taking any treatment to help breathing?	Yes	5
	No	0

*Total scores of ≤18 suggest asthma is the predominant diagnosis, scores of ≥19 suggest COPD.
†Serious enough to keep patient away from work, indoors, at home, or in bed.

indicator for GPs suggests that as a basic requirement, a practice should be able to produce a register of all patients with the condition. Such a register allows easy recall of patients for routine review and an ability to check other related factors such as vaccination status.

Spirometry

Spirometry is the most useful objective measurement of lung function available in primary care. National and international guidelines recommend its use in community settings for both the diagnosis and management of COPD. The availability of low cost, portable, user-friendly machines means that spirometry can now be used as the standard measurement of lung function in the majority of primary care settings and replaces less useful and less informative peak expiratory flow measurements.

Spirometry must be performed by staff who have been trained in the maintenance of the equipment and on how to correctly produce accurate and repeatable measurements. Individuals in the community who perform spirometry should undergo similar training as technicians based at local specialist centres and skills should be updated regularly.

Follow-up of stable COPD in the community

Many patients with COPD will require regular contact with community medical services; those with stable disease may not seek help, but they should be offered a routine review appointment to assess their disease and treatment. Current guidelines suggest that those with mild to moderate disease should be seen at least

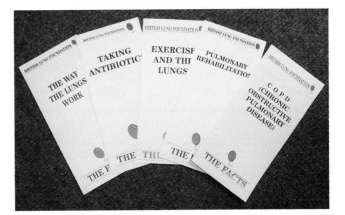

Figure 13.1 All patients should receive written education about COPD and its treatment.

annually, while planned review of those with more severe disease should take place at least twice a year and possibly more frequently as need dictates. Review should also be arranged 4–6 weeks after a change in treatment or within a few weeks of an exacerbation. The following topics should usually be covered:

- Smoking status
- Symptom control
- Treatment regime and concordance
- Signs/symptoms of complications
- Any additional input required
- Examination
- Spirometry
- Assessment of breathlessness (using Medical Research Council (MRC) scale)
- Pulse oximetry if available
- Nutritional state (body mass index (BMI) calculation)
- Mental state; is their evidence of anxiety or depression?
- Vaccination status
- Patient education (such as knowledge of the disease, treatments and inhaler technique; Figure 13.1).

Reviews should take place with those members of the team who specialise in the treatment of COPD and this may include GPs, practice nurses, health visitors, community physiotherapists, community pharmacists, occupational therapists and nurse specialists. Because of the number of team members who may be potentially involved in the care of an individual, it is important that all members of the team have knowledge of the management plan in use and are able to share information with each other. Using one set of electronic records which can be accessed by all relevant healthcare professionals will most easily facilitate this.

Organisation of care at a practice level

The GMS contract for GPs in the United Kingdom includes a set of QOF indicators for COPD. The level at which these indicators are achieved dictates the level of remuneration GPs receive for caring for patients with COPD. In order to achieve targets, many practices have revised their organisation of care in order that accurate, easily accessible records are kept and treatment is optimised for all patients. The QOF does not set out standards for best practice and care, but suggests a minimal level of standard which should be achievable by all well organised practices.

In order to meet the QOF indicators (2009–2010) for COPD, a practice must be able to produce a register of all patients who have been diagnosed with the condition (Figures 13.2 and 13.3). The majority of patients should have had their diagnosis confirmed by spirometry if diagnosed within the last 5 years. All patients should have smoking status recorded annually and advice given/help offered where necessary. In order to meet the minimum standard, the majority of patients should have their forced expiratory volume in one second (FEV_1) recorded and degree of breathlessness assessed using the MRC dyspnoea score each year (Chapter 3). Inhaler technique should be checked (and corrected where necessary) at least annually. The majority of patients must also have been offered influenza vaccine each year; although not specifically outlined in the QOF indicators for COPD 2009–2010, guidelines do recommend that pneumococcal vaccination should be offered. These standards have been easily achieved by the majority

of GPs for some time; however, the need to demonstrate that they are actually met has led to many practices revisiting the way in which care is delivered and recorded.

National strategy

A National Strategy for COPD in England will be published by the Department of Health in 2010. This – the first of its kind in the United Kingdom – is designed to improve diagnosis, support, patient care and education around the disease. Of particular relevance to primary care teams will be the development of a strategy for better identification of undiagnosed and poorly managed cases. The strategy will also focus on helping patients to be dealt with more effectively in the community via development of managed clinical networks and providing effective support and education for both carers and patients to facilitate better understanding and overall care.

Smoking cessation

The GMS contract now rewards practices for recording the smoking status of patients over 15 years of age and for offering smoking cessation support services. Successfully supporting patients in their efforts to give up smoking can help prevent them from developing COPD and facilitate further wide-reaching health benefits. Smoking cessation is also beneficial for patients who have already developed COPD – irrespective of disease severity. Most patients are fully aware of the adverse effects of smoking in general terms, and 'lectures' on problems which may occur in the future are unlikely to be effective in bringing about a change in habit.

It is important to assess patients' readiness to make a change in their behaviour and a useful framework to use as an assessment

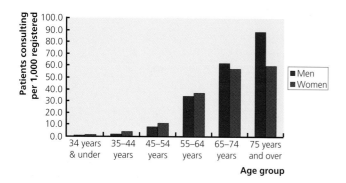

Figure 13.2 Estimated number of patients with COPD in Scotland consulting a general practitioner (GP) or practice nurse at least once in the financial year 2007–2008 per 1,000 patients registered by gender and age group (figure reproduced with permission from http://www.isdscotland.org/isd/3707.html).

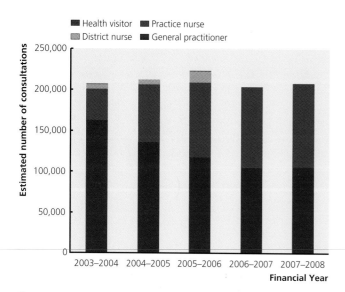

Figure 13.3 Estimated number of consultations by patients with COPD in Scotland in the financial years 2003–2004 to 2007–2008 by staff discipline (figure reproduced with permission from http://www.isdscotland.org/isd/3707.html).

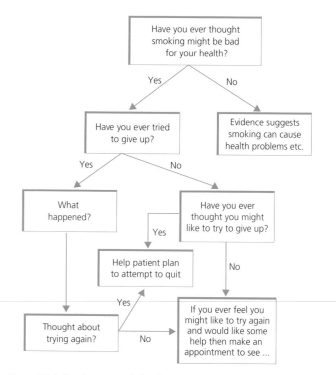

Figure 13.4 Simple structured plan for assessing readiness for an attempt to stop smoking.

tool is the 'States of Change' model (Figure 13.4). This model describes the four stages involved in making a change in behaviour together with maintenance or relapse. Knowing which stage a patient has reached allows more appropriate discussions to take place and an open question such as 'have you ever tried to give up?' allows you to determine where on the model a patient is at any particular time.

Referral for specialist opinion

The decision to refer for a specialist opinion may occur at any stage in the disease. This will also depend on the individual primary care provider's experience, available facilities and confidence in managing COPD. Reasons for specialist referral include

- diagnostic uncertainty,
- severe airflow obstruction,
- marked functional impairment,
- rapidly declining lung function,
- assessment of suitability of domiciliary oxygen in hypoxic patients,
- young age or family history of alpha-1 antitrypsin deficiency,
- persistent symptoms despite apparent adequate therapy,
- frequent exacerbations and infections,
- haemoptysis or suspected lung cancer,
- presence of signs suggestive of cor pulmonale,
- assessment and consideration of specialist treatment such as nebulisers, pulmonary rehabilitation, domiciliary non-invasive ventilation, lung volume reduction surgery, lung transplantation, bullectomy.

Management of stable disease

This is discussed in Chapters 6, 7 and 8.

Management of acute exacerbations

Most acute exacerbations can be successfully managed in the community (Chapter 11). This is usually with 7–14 days of prednisolone 30–40 mg/day, broad-spectrum antibiotics (especially if sputum is more purulent and of greater quantity than usual), regular use of inhaled bronchodilators and other usual inhaled and oral treatments. Some patients may also find short-term use of a nebuliser to deliver bronchodilators of benefit.

The decision to admit a patient to hospital relies on a combination of medical and social factors, which may vary according to the facilities available to the clinician making the decision (Table 13.3). Some exacerbations can also be easily managed in the community following brief assessment at hospital by way of immediate, early or assisted discharge schemes (Chapter 11).

Patients may find a self-management plan useful, which normally gives advice on how to recognise and deal with an exacerbation. The content of a self-management plan will probably vary according to

Table 13.3 Factors to consider when deciding where to most suitably manage a patient with an acute exacerbation of COPD.

Factor	Favours home care	Favours admission
Able to look after themselves	Yes	No
Degree of breathlessness	Mild	Severe
General condition	Good	Worsening
Level of consciousness	Normal	Confused or impaired conscious level
Rate of onset	Gradual	Rapid
Using long-term oxygen therapy	No	Yes
Social circumstances	Good	Less than ideal
Significant co-morbidity, e.g. heart disease, insulin-dependent diabetes	No	Yes
Oxygen saturation	>90%	<90%
Cyanosis	No	Yes
Worsening oedema	No	Yes
Community team available to support care at home if required	Yes	No

the patient population (and indeed individual patients), but should include

- how to recognise an exacerbation;
- what treatment to take and its anticipated duration (antibiotics, oral corticosteroids and increase in bronchodilators);
- whom to contact in an emergency (including out of hours services or the nearest emergency room facility), and how to recognise that they need to do so.

When it is agreed by all health professionals that the final stages of COPD have been reached and that a patient is no longer responsive to medical therapy, palliative care may be offered either in the community or hospice setting (Chapter 14). Palliative care and support should be provided for these patients and carers by the full range of community healthcare team members in the same manner as for any other terminal disease.

Further reading

Chetty M, McKenzie M, Douglas JG, Currie GP. Immediate and early discharge for patients with exacerbations of chronic obstructive pulmonary disease: is their a role in "real-life"? *International Journal of COPD* 2006; **1**: 401–407.

Johannessen A, Omenaas ER, Bakke PS, Gulsvik A. Implications of reversibility testing on prevalence and risk factors for chronic obstructive pulmonary disease: a community study. *Thorax* 2005; **60**: 842–847.

Quality and Outcomes Framework Guidance for GMS Contract 2009/10 http://www.nhsemployers.org/Aboutus/Publications/Documents/QOF_Guidance_2009_final.pdf

http://www.ccq.nl/

http://www.patient.co.uk/health/Chronic-Obstructive-Pulmonary-Disease.htm

http://www.patient.co.uk/health/Smoking-The-Facts.htm

http://clinicalevidence.bmj.com/ceweb/conditions/rdc/1502/copd-standard-ce_patient_leaflet.pdf

CHAPTER 14

Death, Dying and End-of-Life Issues

Gordon Linklater

Roxburghe House, Aberdeen, UK

OVERVIEW

- Chronic obstructive pulmonary disease (COPD) is a life-limiting disease

- Distressing symptoms – such as breathlessness, fatigue, depression and pain – are common in end-stage disease

- Effective symptom management requires a multidisciplinary and holistic approach

- Benzodiazepines and morphine can help relieve persistent breathlessness; when carefully titrated against symptoms, they do not hasten death

- Planning for end-of-life care should happen in parallel with life-prolonging treatments

Palliative care is defined as 'an approach that improves the quality of life of patients and their families, facing the problems associated with life-threatening illness, through the prevention and relief of suffering by means of early identification, assessment and treatment of pain and other problems; physical, psychosocial and spiritual'. This approach requires care to be tailored to the individual needs of patients using the complementary skills of the multidisciplinary team. Palliative care should be available in all care environments, irrespective of whether a diagnosis of cancer has been made.

Chronic obstructive pulmonary disease (COPD) is the most common respiratory disorder which requires palliation of symptoms. Its disease trajectory – usually punctuated by exacerbations resulting in peaks and troughs in levels of functioning and well-being – differs from that of lung cancer and dementia/general frailty (Figure 14.1a,b,c). Nevertheless, patients with end-stage COPD need a structured palliative care programme no less than those with malignant disease.

Maintaining quality of life

Quality of life is difficult to define on an individual basis. In general, health-related quality of life deteriorates as the disease progresses. However, for many patients, particularly those who are aware that they have a life-limiting illness, factors that influence quality of life tend not to be biomedical, but reflect issues of control and

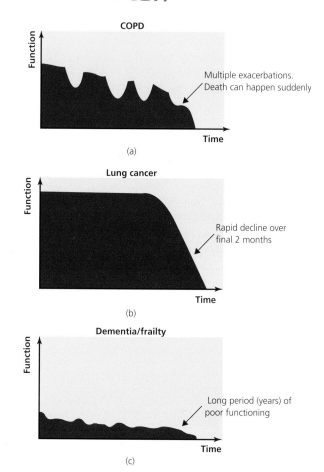

Figure 14.1 Typical disease trajectory in patients with chronic obstructive pulmonary disease (COPD), lung cancer and dementia/general frailty.

interpersonal relationships (Table 14.1). Most patients, therefore, find open and honest discussion about end-of-life issues and involvement in decision-making to be worthwhile and beneficial.

When do patients enter a palliative phase?

Accurately predicting the prognosis of COPD is impossible. Indeed, exacerbations are a common occurrence and it is impossible to know which one will ultimately result in death. These episodic deteriorations can be life threatening, but may also respond to intensive

ABC of COPD, 2nd edition.
Edited by Graeme P. Currie. © 2011 Blackwell Publishing Ltd.

Table 14.1 Factors affecting individual quality of life.

Enhanced by	Diminished by
Maintaining control	Losing independence
Family	Feeling a burden
Hobbies/activities	Lost activities, hobbies, employment
Caring attitude of staff	Pain or fear of pain
Feeling safe/not alone	
Physical environment	

Table 14.2 Predictors of poor prognosis.

General	Factors related to COPD
Weight loss (>10% over 6 months)	FEV$_1$ <30% predicted
Serum albumin <25 g/l	Recurrent hospital admissions (>3 admissions in 12 months for exacerbations)
Multiple co-morbidities	Fulfils long-term oxygen therapy criteria
Declining performance status	Previous non-invasive ventilation for hypercapnic respiratory failure
	Cor pulmonale

COPD, chronic obstructive pulmonary disease; FEV$_1$, forced expiratory volume in one second.

treatment with patients returning to previous levels of health. However, death, when it does happen during an exacerbation, can seem sudden and unexpected. The presence or absence of some clinical features may help guide discussions to some extent (Table 14.2). Unlike many cancers, there is no clear cut-off threshold as to when disease-modifying treatments are no longer appropriate. Instead, a model of care is needed where poor long-term prognosis is acknowledged and symptoms are controlled even while treatments aimed at prolonging life are implemented. However, it is important to strike a pragmatic balance between maintaining a degree of hope for the future and realism about anticipated life-expectancy.

Symptoms

Distressing symptoms – such as breathlessness, fatigue, depression and pain – are common in end-stage disease (Table 14.3). In COPD, particularly during exacerbations, antibiotics, steroids, bronchodilators and non-invasive ventilation (NIV) may all prove useful in relieving symptoms, even when patients are very close to the end of life. Although NIV is generally regarded as a life-saving intervention, it can also be effectively used for palliation. For example, it can be useful in alleviating breathlessness and symptoms related to hypercapnia such as headache. It may also 'buy' the patient and relatives time, whereby outstanding personal, family,

Table 14.3 Prevalence of symptoms in advanced COPD compared to lung cancer.

Symptoms	COPD (%)	Lung cancer (%)
Breathlessness	90	80
Pain	80	85
Fatigue	70	75
Low mood	60	70

COPD, chronic obstructive pulmonary disease.

financial and psychosocial matters can be openly discussed. However, despite maximal medical intervention, patients with advanced COPD often remain highly symptomatic, and other drugs – in particular, benzodiazepines and opiates – play an important role.

Breathlessness

Breathlessness is common in COPD and often associated with fear and panic. Apart from breathlessness due to COPD *per se*, other causes such as anaemia, pulmonary oedema and atrial fibrillation should be considered and managed. Many non-drug strategies such as reassurance, distraction (such as family visits, television, art classes), adapting daily activities, energy conservation, relaxation classes (Figure 14.2) and postural advice (upright, with shoulders supported and relaxed to promote abdominal breathing) are helpful and inexpensive. Some patients find that a moving stream of cool air produced by a bedside fan or an open window can help (Figure 14.3), while supplementary oxygen is useful in the presence

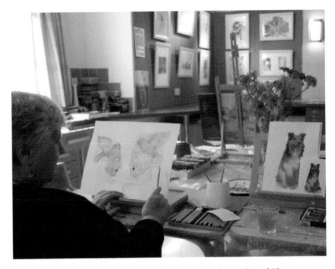

Figure 14.2 Activities and environment can improve quality of life.

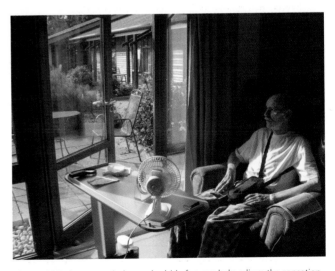

Figure 14.3 An open window or bedside fan can help relieve the sensation of breathlessness.

of hypoxia. For patients with end-stage disease who continue to have troublesome breathlessness despite maximal treatment, a low threshold to starting opioids and/or benzodiazepines should exist (Boxes 14.1 and 14.2). Careful titration of these drugs will not hasten death.

Box 14.1 Use of opioids in end-stage COPD

- Reduce the sensation of breathlessness.
- Initially use oral morphine (e.g. Oramorph or Sevredol 2.5 mg) as required.
- Long-acting morphine preparations may be useful to control 'background' breathlessness (e.g. MST 10 mg twice daily).

Box 14.2 Use of benzodiazepines in end-stage COPD

- Useful for breathlessness associated with anxiety.
- Can be used alone or with opioids.
- Initially use lorazepam (0.5 mg sublingually) as required.
- Patients with persistent anxiety/breathlessness may benefit from more regular dosing from a longer acting benzodiazepine (e.g. diazepam 2–5 mg two to three times daily).

Pain

Pain has a similar prevalence in both COPD and lung cancer. Regular paracetamol and non-steroidal anti-inflammatory drugs with the addition of regular morphine for moderate to severe pain are the mainstays of treatment. The use of heat pads, cold pads and TENS (transcutaneous electrical nerve stimulation) machines are often useful (Figure 14.4). Different pain types may also respond to different treatment modalities; for example, for neuropathic pain consider tricyclic antidepressants or anticonvulsants, and for an osteoporotic rib fracture consider an intercostal nerve block.

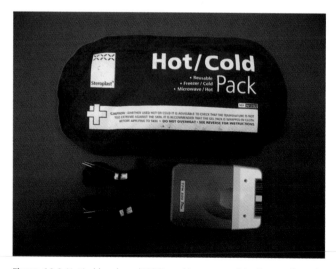

Figure 14.4 Hot/cold pads and TENS machines are useful adjuvants for pain control.

Fatigue

Fatigue is highly prevalent in all life-limiting illnesses. Reversible underlying causes should be sought and treated where possible (for example, anaemia, hypothyroidism, poor sleep hygiene and excessive sedative medications). Drug treatments for fatigue are ineffective, although occupational therapist and physiotherapist interventions can be invaluable (e.g. graded exercise programmes, energy conservation techniques, provision of aids for activities of daily living) in this respect.

Depression and anxiety

Depression is underdiagnosed and undertreated in patients with advanced COPD. Untreated depression makes dealing with other physical or psychosocial issues more difficult. While many symptoms of depression can be found in advanced physical disease (fatigue, loss of appetite and disturbed sleep), feelings of worthlessness or inappropriate guilt are highly suggestive of an underlying depressive disorder. Moreover, a good screening test is simply, 'are you depressed?'. Several classes of antidepressants are available. Examples include the following:

- Sertraline (initial dose 50 mg at night, titrated by 50 mg every 2 weeks to a maximum dose of 200 mg once daily) – may cause gastrointestinal upset.
- Amitriptyline (initial dose 10–25 mg at night, titrated cautiously to 75–150 mg at night) – useful if sedation is required or neuropathic pain is a problem; anticholinergic side-effects commonly limit dose titration, particularly in the elderly.
- Mirtazapine (initial dose 15 mg at night, titrated by 15 mg a week to 45 mg at night) – useful if patient is anxious; may also help neuropathic pain and stimulate appetite.

Anxiety is common near end of life, and is exacerbated by feeling out of control or other significant symptoms, particularly breathlessness. Benzodiazepines are the mainstays of drug treatment, although sedative antidepressants may also be useful.

Advanced care planning

Similar proportions of patients with COPD and lung cancer would opt for 'comfort care' over 'life-prolonging care', yet those with COPD are less likely to have end-of-life discussions with their doctor. Discussion about the dying process allows patients to choose what arrangements should be made to manage the final stages of their illness, and to attend to personal and other concerns considered important towards end of life.

Decisions about withholding or withdrawing life-prolonging treatment can be difficult and distressing. However, it is important to be aware of the following:

- Competent adults may decide to refuse treatment even where refusal may result in harm to themselves or in their own death; clinicians are bound to respect a competent refusal of treatment.

- Where an adult patient has become incompetent, a refusal of treatment made when the patient was competent must be respected, provided it is clearly applicable to the present circumstances and there is no reason to believe that the patient had changed his/her mind.
- There is no obligation to give treatment that is futile and burdensome; in the context of end-stage COPD, cardiopulmonary resuscitation has a negligible success rate.
- Final responsibility rests with the clinician to decide what treatments are clinically indicated; these should be provided subject to a competent patient's consent or, in the case of an incompetent patient, any known views of that patient prior to becoming incapacitated and taking account of the views offered by the family.
- Family members/carers/'next of kin' do not have decision-making rights or responsibilities for treatment consent/refusal (unless the patient has designated a proxy decision maker, e.g. a power of attorney).

Advance refusal of treatment

Advance refusals of treatment – also known as 'living wills' or 'advance directives' – are legal documents that allow patients to indicate their preferences for care, should they no longer be able to make decisions due to illness or incapacity. An advance refusal of treatment can specify that under certain circumstances the patient can withdraw consent for life-supporting interventions. Such a refusal is binding, as long as it clearly relates to the current circumstances. A patient can make an advanced statement of preferences for treatment and care, but this statement cannot demand treatment that is deemed clinically inappropriate. An advance refusal may be invalid if:

- it does not relate to current circumstances;
- there is reason to doubt authenticity;
- it is felt that there was duress;
- there is doubt as to the person's state of mind (at the time of signing).

If a patient is considering an advance refusal of treatment he/she should be encouraged to discuss its contents with family/carers and ensure that a copy is placed in his/her medical records. Legal advice, to help draft the form and provide a witness signature, may also be useful.

End-of-life care

Where the rapid progression of a patient's end-stage condition is likely, and death is considered an inevitable outcome, it is important to ensure that terminal care needs are identified and met appropriately. This should include consideration of wishes regarding the appropriate place for receiving care, which may affect treatment options available (e.g. home, care home, cottage hospital or hospital), and the need for religious, spiritual, family or other personal support.

If patients are admitted to hospital, unnecessary interventions should also stop (e.g. regular venepuncture, arterial blood gases, routine monitoring of vital signs) and the appropriateness of medications (e.g. statins, anti-platelet drugs, heparin, proton pump inhibitors, etc.) should frequently be reviewed. The most common symptoms in the terminal phase are pain, breathlessness, anxiety/agitation and copious respiratory secretions ('death rattle'). In anticipating these symptoms, 'as-required' medications should be prescribed early to allow rapid symptom control (Box 14.3). If the patient is at home, arrangements will be needed to ensure that staff are available to administer such treatments over a 24-hour period if necessary.

Box 14.3 Drugs used in terminal care

- Morphine 2.5 mg* subcutaneous as required for pain or breathlessness
- Midazolam 2.5 mg subcutaneous as required for agitation or breathlessness
- Hyoscine hydrobromide 400 μg subcutaneous as required for respiratory secretions (Hyoscine butylbromide and glycopyrronium are non-sedative alternatives.)

*if opioid naive. If not opioid naïve, the dose should be half the oral 'breakthrough' dose of immediate release morphine i.e. Oramorph or Sevredol.

Further reading

Claessens MT, Lynn J, Zhong Z et al. Dying with lung cancer or chronic obstructive pulmonary disease: insights from SUPPORT. *Journal of American Geriatric Society* 2000; **48**: S146–S153.

Edmonds P, Karlsen S, Khan S, Addington-Hall J. A comparison of the palliative care needs of patients dying from chronic respiratory diseases and lung cancer. *Palliative Medicine* 2001; **35**: 287–295.

Elkington H, White P, Addington-Hall J, Higgs R, Edmonds P. The healthcare needs of chronic obstructive pulmonary disease patients in the last year of life. *Palliative Medicine* 2005; **19**: 485–491.

Fallon M, Hanks G. *ABC of Palliative Care*, 2nd edn. Blackwell Publishing, Oxford, 2006.

Gore JM, Brophy CJ, Greenstone MA. How well do we care for patients with end stage chronic obstructive pulmonary disease (COPD)? A comparison of palliative care and quality of life in COPD and lung cancer. *Thorax* 2000; **55**: 1000–1006.

Rocker G, Horton R, Currow D, Goodridge D, Young J, Booth S. Palliation of dyspnoea in advanced COPD: revisiting a role for opioids. *Thorax* 2009; **64**: 910–915.

http://www.goldstandardsframework.nhs.uk/

http://www.gmc-uk.org/guidance/current/library/witholding_lifeprolonging_guidance.asp

CHAPTER 15

Future Treatments

Peter J. Barnes

National Heart and Lung Institute, Imperial College London, London, UK

OVERVIEW

- Effective drug development in chronic obstructive pulmonary disease (COPD) is hindered because of a variety of methodological issues relating to clinical trials

- Once-daily long-acting inhaled bronchodilators (alone or in combination) may become the mainstay of pharmacological treatment in the future

- More effective smoking cessation strategies are in varying degrees of development

- Specially designed anti-inflammatory agents and mediator antagonists may play a role in the future

Current therapy for the treatment of COPD is often less than ideal and fails to reduce the relentless decline in lung function that leads to increasing symptoms, disability and exacerbations or reduce mortality. Many pharmaceutical companies are therefore seeking more effective therapies that may control or even reverse the underlying disease process.

The continuing challenge of drug development

There are several reasons why drug development in COPD has proved to be difficult. For example,

- the molecular and cell biology of COPD is still poorly understood, although there have been important advances and increasing research in this area, leading to the identification of new therapeutic targets;
- animal models of COPD for early drug testing (usually smoking mice) are unsatisfactory as they do not mimic all the features of the disease, particularly small airway fibrosis and exacerbations;
- there is uncertainty about which biomarkers in blood, sputum or breath may predict clinical efficacy;
- there are methodological uncertainties about how best to evaluate drugs for COPD in the long term, although there is increasing

interest in patient-reported outcome measures, since changes in FEV_1 poorly reflect clinical improvements;
- many patients with COPD have important co-morbidities – such as ischaemic heart disease, cardiac failure, hypertension and diabetes mellitus – which may exclude them from clinical trials of new therapies and therefore create uncertainty regarding the usefulness of some drugs in 'real-life'.

However, despite all of these issues, progress is underway and several new classes of drugs are now in the pre-clinical and clinical stages of development.

New bronchodilators

The mainstay of current drug therapy in COPD consists of long-acting bronchodilators. A long-acting anticholinergic (tiotropium once daily) and long-acting β_2-agonists (salmeterol and formoterol twice daily) are the preferred first-line agents in symptomatic individuals with established disease (Box 15.1). There are several new once-daily ('ultra-long-acting') β_2-agonists, such as indacaterol, for use in patients with COPD (Figure 15.1). New once-daily long-acting muscarinic antagonists, such as glycopyrronium and aclidinium, are also undergoing clinical trials. Ultra-long-acting β_2-agonists and long-acting anti-muscarinics appear to have additive bronchodilator effects, so that fixed combination inhalers containing both classes of drug are also in varying stages of development. Moreover, dual function molecules that have long-acting anti-muscarinic and long-acting β_2-agonist activity are being evaluated in clinical trials. Although there has been a search for novel classes of bronchodilators – such as potassium channel openers – these have proved to be less effective than established bronchodilators and exhibit more adverse effects.

Combination inhalers that contain an inhaled corticosteroid plus a long-acting β_2-agonist are commonly prescribed for patients with more advanced COPD. Both salmeterol plus fluticasone (Seretide) and formoterol plus budesonide (Symbicort) are more effective than their separate constituents as monotherapy, and are indicated in patients with more advanced airflow obstruction ($FEV_1 < 50\%$ predicted) who have frequent exacerbations (more than two per year). Fixed combination inhalers containing a long-acting corticosteroid and an ultra-long-acting β_2-agonist are now in development for once-daily dosing.

ABC of COPD, 2nd edition.
Edited by Graeme P. Currie. © 2011 Blackwell Publishing Ltd.

Box 15.1 **Current and future long-acting bronchodilators for the treatment of COPD**

Long-acting β₂-agonists

- Salmeterol (twice daily)*
- Formoterol (once daily)*
- Indacaterol (once daily)
- Carmoterol (once daily)
- Vilanterol (once daily)
- Olodaterol (once daily)

Long-acting anticholinergics

- Tiotropium bromide (once daily)*
- Glycopyrronium bromide (once daily)
- Aclidinium bromide (once or twice daily)
- Daratropium bromide (once daily)

Combination inhalers

- Salmeterol/fluticasone propionate (Seretide: twice daily)*
- Formoterol/budesonide (Symbicort: twice daily)*
- Vilanterol/fluticasone furoate (once daily)
- Indacaterol/mometasone furoate (once daily)
- Indacaterol/glycopyrronium bromide (once daily)
- Olodaterol/tiotropium bromide (once daily)

Muscarinic antagonist/β-agonist (MABA)

- GSK-961081

* Already licensed for use in COPD.

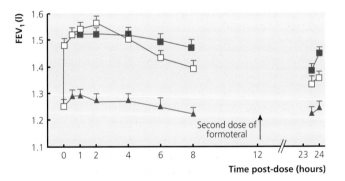

Figure 15.1 Effect of the ultra-long-acting β₂-agonist indacaterol (■) compared to the twice-daily long-acting beta agonist (LABA) formoterol (□) and placebo (▲) on forced expiratory volume in one second (FEV_1) in COPD patients. Figure produced with permission from Beier J *et al. Pulmonary Pharmacology & Therapeutics* 2009; **22**: 492–496.

More effective smoking cessation strategies

Cigarette smoking is the major cause of COPD in the United Kingdom and quitting at most stages of the disease reduces disease progression. Smoking cessation is therefore an integral part of management, although current cessation strategies have had only limited long-term success. The most effective current aid to smoking cessation is the partial nicotine agonist varenicline, which targets the $\alpha_4\beta_2$ nicotinic acetylcholine receptor (Figure 15.2). Although varenicline

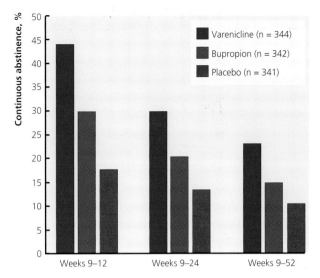

Figure 15.2 Effect of varenicline compared to bupropion and placebo on smoking cessation in normal subjects. Figure produced with permission from Jorenby DE *et al. JAMA* 2006; **296**: 56–63. Copyright © (2006) American Medical Association. All rights reserved.

is more effective than bupropion and nicotine replacement therapy, it still only achieves a quit rate of approximately 20% in 1 year and adverse effects – such as nausea and depression – may limit its use. Another approach which may have longer term benefits is the development of a vaccine against nicotine, which stimulates the production of antibodies that bind nicotine, meaning that it is unable to enter the brain. Several nicotine vaccines are currently undergoing evaluation in clinical trials as are several other pharmacological approaches (Box 15.2).

Box 15.2 **Current and future drugs for smoking cessation**

Current therapies

- Nicotine replacement therapy
- Bupropion
- Varenicline ($\alpha_4\beta_2$ partial nicotine agonist)

Future therapies

- Cannabinoid CB_1-receptor antagonists (e.g. rimonabant)
- $GABA_B$ antagonists
- Dopamine D_3 antagonists
- Nicotine vaccination (e.g. nic-Vax)

Treating pulmonary inflammation

COPD is characterised by chronic inflammation – particularly involving the small airways and lung parenchyma. The pattern of inflammation is different from that of asthma, with a predominance of macrophages, neutrophils and cytotoxic T lymphocytes and different inflammatory mediators being involved. In sharp contrast to asthma, the inflammation is largely resistant to the anti-inflammatory effects of corticosteroids, which has prompted the search for alternative anti-inflammatory therapies. Indeed, better understanding of the underlying mechanisms in COPD has led to the development of several potential therapeutic targets.

Mediator antagonists

Many mediators – including lipid mediators and cytokines – are implicated in the pathophysiology of COPD. Inhibiting specific mediators, by receptor antagonists or synthesis inhibitors, is a relatively easy approach. However, doing so is unlikely to produce effective drugs, since so many mediators with similar effects are involved. Currently, several mediator antagonists are in clinical development. This is based on research demonstrating that the particular mediator level is increased in COPD, and in turn mimics some of the effects observed in COPD (Box 15.3). Anti-tumour necrosis factor antibodies are currently used to treat patients with severe rheumatoid arthritis and inflammatory bowel disease, but have been ineffective in COPD and may be associated with an increased risk of pneumonia and lung cancer. An interleukin-8 blocking antibody also appears to be largely ineffective. More promising strategies are small molecule antagonists of the chemokine receptor CXCR2, which mediates the effects of interleukin-8 and related chemokines. Preliminary studies show that these drugs reduce neutrophilic inflammation in sputum in normal subjects after endotoxin and ozone challenge, and are currently being evaluated in clinical trials.

Box 15.3 **Mediator antagonists for potential use in COPD**

Mediator	Major effect	Inhibitor
Leukotriene B_4	Neutrophil chemotaxis	BLT_1 -receptor antagonists (e.g. BIIL284) 5'-lipoxygenase inhibitors
Interleukin-8	Neutrophil chemotaxis	Blocking antibodies (e.g. ABX-IL8) CXCR2 antagonists (e.g. Sch527123)
Interleukin-1β	Amplifying inflammation	Blocking antibodies (e.g. canakinumab)
Interleukin-6	Amplifying inflammation	Blocking receptor antibody (e.g. tocilizumab)
Tumour necrosis factor-α	Amplifying inflammation	Blocking antibodies (e.g. infliximab) Soluble receptors (e.g. etanercept)
Epidermal growth factor	Mucus hypersecretion	EGFR kinase inhibitors (e.g. gefitinib)
Oxidative stress	Amplifying inflammation Steroid resistance	Antioxidants (e.g. superoxide dismutase analogues)
Nitrative stress	Steroid resistance	Inducible NO synthase inhibitors (e.g. GSK-274150)

Oxidative stress is increased in COPD, particularly as the disease becomes more advanced and during exacerbations. Oxidative stress amplifies inflammation and may result in corticosteroid resistance, and is therefore a potentially important target for future therapies. Current antioxidants are not very effective, but more potent and stable antioxidants – such as analogues of superoxide dismutase and activators of the transcription factor Nrf2, which regulates several antioxidant genes – are now in development.

Protease inhibitors

Several proteases such as elastases – which are implicated in alveolar destruction – are a target for therapy in patients with COPD with marked emphysema. Proteases may be inhibited by giving endogenous antiproteases, such as α1-antitrypsin, or by small molecule protease inhibitors (Box 15.4). However, no clinical studies have yet demonstrated that these approaches have any beneficial effect.

Box 15.4 **Protease inhibitors for potential use in COPD**

Protease inhibitor	Endogenous antiprotease	Small molecule
Neutrophil elastase	α1-Antitrypsin Secretory leukoprotease inhibitor Elafin	ONO-5046
Cathepsins	Cystatins	Cysteine protease inhibitor
Matrix metalloproteinases MMP-9	Tissue inhibitors of MMPs TIMP-1	Marimastat MMP-9/12 selective (e.g. AZ11557272)

New anti-inflammatory treatments

Since corticosteroids are ineffective in reducing the inflammation found in COPD, alternative anti-inflammatory therapies are needed. The most promising new anti-inflammatory agents are phosphodiesterase (PDE)-4 inhibitors. These orally active drugs increase cyclic adenosine monophosphate concentrations in inflammatory cells and exhibit a broad-spectrum of anti-inflammatory effects. Although effective in animal models of COPD, PDE-4 inhibitors (such roflumilast) have had limited success because of adverse effects – particularly nausea, diarrhoea and weight loss. However, recent large randomised placebo-controlled studies of patients with COPD have shown that treatment with roflumilast reduces exacerbations and improves lung function over 1 year, and provides benefit when added to long-acting bronchodilators (Figure 15.3). More selective inhibitors (PDE-4B inhibitors) and inhaled administration of these drugs are currently being investigated to circumvent the problem of adverse effects. Several other broad-spectrum anti-inflammatory therapies are currently under investigation (Box 15.5), although most of these are likely to be associated with adverse effects when given systemically, suggesting that inhaled administration may be required.

Corticosteroid resistance is one of the typical features of COPD. An alternative therapeutic strategy is therefore to reverse the molecular mechanism of this resistance, which appears to be due to reduced expression and activity of the nuclear enzyme histone deacetylase (HDAC)-2. This can be achieved *in vitro* by theophylline, which acts as an HDAC activator, or by inhibiting oxidative/nitrative stress. Other therapeutic strategies

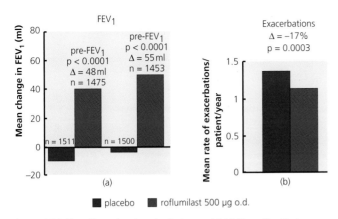

Figure 15.3 The effect of a phosphodiesterase-4 inhibitor roflumilast (500 mg orally once daily) on forced expiratory volume in one second (FEV_1) (a) and on acute exacerbations (b) in patients with COPD. Figure adapted with permission from Roflumilast in symptomatic chronic obstructive pulmonary disease: two randomised clinical trials. Calverley PM, Rabe KF, Goehring UM *et al. Lancet* 2009; **374**: 685–694.

to reverse steroid resistance include macrolides, nortriptyline and phosphoinositide-3-kinase-δ inhibitors, all of which restore HDAC2 levels (Box 15.6).

Box 15.5 **Novel anti-inflammatory treatments for COPD**

- Phosphodiesterase-4 inhibitors (e.g. roflumilast)
- p38 Mitogen-activated protein kinase inhibitors (e.g. SB-681323)
- Nuclear factor-κB inhibitors (e.g. AS602868)
- Phosphoinositide-3-kinase-γ and δ inhibitors
- Peroxisome proliferator-activated receptor-γ (PPAR-γ) agonists (e.g. rosiglitazone)
- Adhesion molecule inhibitors (e.g. bimosiamose)
- Non-antibiotic macrolides
- Resveratrol analogues

Box 15.6 **Reversal of steroid resistance in COPD**

- Theophylline (HDAC activator)
- Nortriptyline (HDAC activator)
- Phosphoinositide-3-kinase-δ inhibitors (HDAC activators)
- HDAC2-selective activators
- Antioxidants
- Inducible NO synthase inhibitors
- Peroxynitrite scavengers

Lung repair

COPD is a largely irreversible disease process, but it is possible that enhanced repair of the damage might restore lung function in the future. There has been particular interest in retinoic acid, which is able to reverse experimental emphysema in rats. However, this is unlikely to work in humans, whose lungs do not have the regenerative capacity of that found in rats; to date, human studies have been negative. Another approach being explored is the use of stem cells in an attempt to regenerate alveolar type 1 cells.

Route of delivery

Drugs for airway diseases are traditionally given by inhalation. However, inhaler devices usually target larger airways that are predominantly involved in asthma, while elderly patients or those with musculoskeletal problems may have difficulty in using conventional inhaler devices. In COPD, the inflammation is mainly found in the small airways and lung parenchyma, in turn suggesting that devices that deliver drugs more peripherally may be of greater benefit. A more systemic approach facilitated by oral drug delivery is therefore an attractive option, as the lung periphery would be targeted. Oral therapies could also have an impact upon systemic complications that often arise in patients with severe disease, although this would carry an increased risk of adverse effects. An alternative approach is targeted drug delivery by exploiting specific cell uptake mechanisms in target cells, such as macrophages.

Further reading

Barnes PJ. Emerging pharmacotherapies for COPD. *Chest* 2008; **134**: 1278–1286.

Cazzola M, Macnee W, Martinez FJ *et al.* Outcomes for COPD pharmacological trials: from lung function to biomarkers. *European Respiratory Journal* 2008; **31**: 416–469.

Cazzola M, Matera MG. Emerging inhaled bronchodilators: an update. *European Respiratory Journal* 2009; **34**: 757–769.

Fabbri LM, Calverley PM, Izquierdo-Alonso JL *et al.* Roflumilast in moderate-to-severe chronic obstructive pulmonary disease treated with long-acting bronchodilators: two randomised clinical trials. *Lancet* 2009; **374**: 695–703.

Hansel TT, Barnes PJ. New drugs for exacerbations of chronic obstructive pulmonary disease. *Lancet* 2009; **374**: 744–755.

Tashkin DP, Murray RP. Smoking cessation in chronic obstructive pulmonary disease. *Respiratory Medicine* 2009; **103**: 963–974.

Index

Note: Page numbers in *italics* refer to figures and those in **bold** refer to tables and box matters